NewHope

FOR COUPLES WITH

Infertility Problems

Other Books in Prima's NEW HOPE Series

New Hope for People with Alzheimer's and Their Caregivers

New Hope for People with Bipolar Disorder

New Hope for People with Borderline Personality Disorder

New Hope for People with Depression

New Hope for People with Diabetes

New Hope for People with Fibromyalgia

New Hope for People with Lupus

New Hope for People with Weight Problems

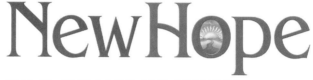

New Hope

FOR COUPLES WITH

Infertility
Problems

Theresa Foy DiGeronimo

Foreword and Medical Review by
Paul R. Gindoff, M.D.

PRIMA PUBLISHING

Published by Prima Publishing, Roseville, California. Member of the Crown Publishing Group, a division of Random House, Inc.

PRIMA PUBLISHING and colophon are trademarks of Random House, Inc., registered with the United States Patent and Trademark Office.

In order to protect their privacy, the names of some individuals cited in this book have been changed.

Warning—Disclaimer

This book is not intended to provide medical advice and is sold with the understanding that the publisher and the author are not liable for the misconception or misuse of information provided. The author and Random House, Inc., shall have neither liability nor responsibility to any person or entity with respect to any loss, damage, or injury caused or alleged to be caused directly or indirectly by the information contained in this book or the use of any products mentioned. Readers should not use any of the products discussed in this book without the advice of a medical professional.

Interior design by Peri Poloni, Knockout Design
Illustrations by Laurie Baker-McNeile

Library of Congress Cataloging-in-Publication Data
DiGeronimo, Theresa Foy
 New hope for couples with infertility problems : your friendly, authoritative guide to the latest in traditional and complementary solutions / Theresa Foy DiGeronimo.
   p. cm.— (New hope)
 Includes bibliographical references and index.
 ISBN 0-7615-2563-7
 1. Infertility 2. Fertility, Human. 3. Human reproductive technology. I. Title. II. Series.

RC889 .D56 2002
616.6'9206—dc21   2002070518

02 03 04 05 DD 10 9 8 7 6 5 4 3 2 1
Printed in the United States of America

First Edition

Visit us online at www.primapublishing.com

Contents

Foreword by Paul R. Gindoff, M.D.   *vii*

Acknowledgments   *ix*

1. An Overview of Infertility   1

2. Diagnosis of Infertility: Getting Some Answers   35

3. Basic Fertility Tips and Complementary and Alternative Medicine   73

4. Medical Infertility Treatments 131

5. Infertility Options: Donor Eggs/Sperm, Surrogate Parenting, Adoption, and Nonparenting   173

6. The Mind, the Body, and Infertility   213

7. A Future Wrapped in High Hopes and Controversy   245

Appendix: Resources   *285*

Notes   *289*

Glossary   *299*

Index   *313*

Foreword

A S A PRACTITIONER in reproductive endocrinology and fertility treatments for over 15 years, I have acquired a great deal of knowledge from my patients. They have taught me how deep the desire to procreate runs, how tenacious one can be in the struggle, and how euphoric one can be when the dream of conception is realized. I have also witnessed the courage and resilience of couples involved in unsuccessful attempts to conceive and appreciate the value of medical innovation, adoption, and resolution in this process.

Decades ago, the rule of thirds was coined in reproductive medicine. This rule indicated that one-third of couples who sought help for infertility problems would conceive because of focused medical treatment, one-third of these couples would conceive regardless of what treatment is done, and one-third would not conceive. The good news is that with the scientific and technological breakthroughs of the last two decades, we've reduced the last category from one-third to roughly one-eighth. Infertility, then, can more appropriately be thought of as "conception delayed." After all, the majority of couples will eventually conceive.

However, despite the new technology and the best intentions on the part of all involved, a significant number of couples will not achieve their goal. This may be the first major disappointment in many of these couples' lives, requiring support, understanding, and coping skills beyond anything they've confronted before.

The challenges to those facing compromised fertility or conception delay are experienced on physical, psychological, emotional, social, and even spiritual fronts. Making the transition through a crisis of infertility is the true measure of success for the individual. Regardless of the outcome, maintaining the integrity of the individuals involved and rediscovering the wonders of living are paramount.

In *New Hope for Couples with Infertility Problems*, author Theresa DiGeronimo develops a comprehensive foundation and resource for all those facing this profound ordeal. Basic biology, advanced genetics, reproductive physiology, medical education and treatment, emotional support and healing, innovative support and alternative therapies, environmental effects, adoption, nonparenting, and more are defined and explored. The goal of this book is to provide comprehensive information to help achieve success in the struggle with infertility. The chapters are well organized, comprehensive, and comprehensible without requiring a degree in biomedical sciences. It makes for an excellent source of information and a resource for planning.

I am glad that you have found this book to use as a resource and guide. May it bring you the fortune you seek.

Paul R. Gindoff, M.D., professor and director
of the Division of Reproductive Endocrinology,
Fertility, and IVF at The George Washington
University Medical Center in Washington, D.C.

Acknowledgments

A DEBT OF gratitude and thanks is due to all the professionals who willingly shared their expertise to make this book as accurate and up-to-date as possible: Gary S. Berger, M.D., Chapel Hill Tubal Reversal Center, Chapel Hill, North Carolina; Keith Blackwell, M.D., Ph.D., Center for Blood Research, Boston, Massachusetts; Melanie Blum, Esq., Tustin, California; Brenda J. Boykin, Washington, D.C.; Hannah Bradford, M.Ac., Center for Integrative Medicine at George Washington University Medical Center, Washington, D.C.; Brian Clement, Hippocrates Health Institute, West Palm Beach, Florida; Serafina Corsell, M.D., New York, New York; Peter Degnan, M.D., Equinox Health and Healing, Portsmouth, New Hampshire; Anna Delury, Studio City, California; Robin Dipasquale, N.D., chair, Botanical Medicine Department, Bastyr University, Kenmore, Washington; Alice Domar, Ph.D., Division of Behavioral Medicine, Harvard Medical School, Boston, Massachusetts; Jean Fourcroy, M.D., Ph.D., Bethesda, Maryland; Peter Gibbs, M.A., L.M.F.T., director of the Center for Adoption Research at the University of Massachusetts; Paul R. Gindoff, M.D., professor and director, Division of Reproductive Endocrinology, Fertility, and IVF, George Washington University Medical Center, Washington, D.C.; Neil F. Goodman, M.D., University of Miami School of Medicine; Clifford Kearns, D.C., Schaumburg, Illinois; Ed Madara, Cedar Knolls, New Jersey; James Madden, M.D., Presbyterian Hospital of Dallas, Texas; John Pan, M.D., director of the

Center for Integrative Medicine, George Washington University Medical Center, Washington, D.C.; Mark Perloe, M.D., medical director, Georgia Reproductive Specialists, Atlanta, Georgia; Steven Petak, M.D., Texas Institute for Reproductive Medicine and Endocrinology, Houston, Texas; Nataly Pluta P.T., Y.T., Pluta Movement Therapeutics, Del Mar, California; Veronica A. Ravnikar, M.D., director of the Division of Reproductive Endocrinology at University of Massachusetts Memorial Medical Center; Scott Roseff, M.D., director, W.E. C.A.R.E., West Orange, New Jersey; Jane Rosenthal, M.D., Columbia Presbyterian Medical Center, New York, New York; David Sable, M.D., Jacques Cohen, Ph.D., and Eric Seaman, M.D., Saint Barnabas Hospital, Livingston, New Jersey; Christina Schlank, Los Angeles, California; Jim Shrybman, Takoma Park, Maryland; Mengda Shu, Center for Integrative Medicine, George Washington University Medical Center, Washington, D.C.; Eric Scott Sills, M.D., Georgia Reproductive Specialists, Atlanta, Georgia; Mary Sullivan, M.S.W., RESOLVE of Illinois; Larry and Belinda Wurn, Clear Passage Therapies, Inc., Gainesville, Florida; and Rebecca Wynsome, N.D., Water's Edge Natural Health Services, Seattle, Washington.

Special thanks also to those who shared their personal experiences: Lisa, Dipak and Penny, Sue and Bob, Theresa, Melinda, Maryann, Rosamunda, Clara, Angela, Susan, Traci, Alice, Leza, Eileen, Jenny, Brenda and Doane, and Erin.

I would also like to thank my helpful and competent editors: Jamie Miller and Marjorie Lery.

CHAPTER 1

An Overview of Infertility

ARE YOU OR your partner infertile? If you have been having sex for over 1 year without any form of contraception (such as birth control pills, diaphragm, condoms, or rhythm method) and you have not gotten pregnant, or if you have had a series of miscarriages, infertility may be the problem. If this is true in your case, don't despair! Based on medical evidence, there is much hope that you can become a parent. After all, infertility is not the same thing as sterility—the inability to conceive a child under any circumstance. Often, a diagnosis of infertility just means delayed conception and that becoming a parent will be a challenge—one that can often be met and overcome.

Steven M. Petak, M.D., associate at the Texas Institute for Reproductive Medicine and Endocrinology in Houston, knows how quickly the word *infertility* can throw a couple into a life crisis, but he remains optimistic. When a couple comes to him with their hearts aching with disappointment, he tells them that relatively simple initial steps often result in pregnancy, such as using basal body temperature charts and correcting underlying hormonal problems. "The chances for pregnancy have never been better than they are now for nearly all women, even when simple solutions don't work," says Dr. Petak. "Assisted reproductive technologies are dramatically improving the chances for pregnancy in women with tubal disease, severe ovulatory dysfunction, and low sperm counts in the spouse. Even in women with ovarian failure, egg donation can be used to achieve pregnancy."

> ## What Exactly Is Infertility?
>
> *Infertility* is the inability to conceive after a year of unprotected intercourse in women under 35, or after 6 months in women over 35, or the inability to carry a pregnancy to a live birth.

This is good news for all couples dealing with the uncertainties of infertility. Of course, the reasons for reproductive problems vary from person to person, and the details of your infertility are personal and unique. But in all cases, the basic reason for infertility lies somewhere within the intricate process of getting sperm to find and fertilize the egg, and then having the egg implant and develop in the uterus. To help you better understand how this process happens (and sometimes doesn't happen), this chapter will explore infertility statistics, the male and female roles in the process of conception, the history of our medical knowledge of fertility and infertility, and the causes of male and female infertility.

THE LONG JOURNEY TO CONCEPTION

We all know how it works—through intercourse, the male sperm meets and fertilizes the female egg, and a child is conceived. When the process works, few couples question the details of how conception happens. But when it doesn't work, you may be more curious to know exactly how the sperm and the egg are supposed to get together in the right place at the right time. This section will give you a brief biology lesson on human conception and fertility. If you are already familiar with the basic terms and pieces of anatomy involved in conception, feel free to skip this section, but if you are just beginning your search for answers, pay close attention. This information will help you better understand much of the information that is to follow later in the book.

The Female's Role

Having a regular monthly menstrual cycle is important in evaluating a woman's level of fertility, but it's only the beginning. For the male's sperm to find its way to the woman's egg, the woman's reproductive organs must allow the sperm to move from the vagina through the cervix and into a fallopian tube. Her tubes must be healthy and be able to help the sperm get to the egg. In addition, the woman must produce a healthy egg and must release the egg from one of her ovaries and have it picked up by the adjacent fallopian tube. The tube must be open so that the egg, after fertilization, can find its way into the uterus. Her reproductive system must then protect and nourish the egg in the uterus.

All parts of the female reproductive system must be healthy for this chain of events to happen. The parts and terms you should be familiar with are illustrated in figures 1.1 and 1.2. They include the following:

- The *vagina* is a muscular, 4-inch-long canal that provides an exit for menstrual blood and an entrance for *semen* (the fluid containing the male sperm).

- The *cervix* is an inch long and is found at the top of the vagina. This is the entrance to the *uterus*. The cervix produces mucus that prevents bacteria and other organisms present in the vagina from entering the uterus. However, just before the time of ovulation (when the egg is released from the ovary) the cervical mucus changes to allow sperm to swim freely by and into the uterus on its way to the fallopian tubes.

- The *ovaries* are two almond-sized structures that are stocked with a lifetime of eggs at birth. No new eggs are formed during the woman's lifetime. Each month, a substance called follicle-stimulating hormone (FSH) is secreted by a woman's pituitary gland, signaling the ovaries to mature an egg follicle (a fluid-filled capsule). When one, or sometimes two, of these

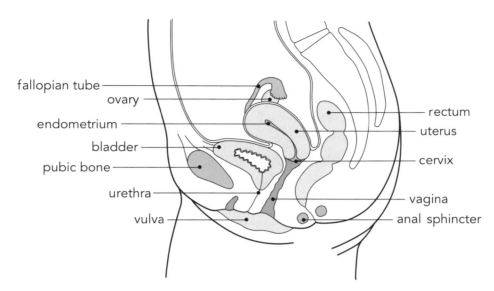

fallopian tube

ovary

endometrium

bladder

pubic bone

urethra

vulva

rectum

uterus

cervix

vagina

anal sphincter

Figure 1.1—*Female Pelvis Cross-Section*

follicles have reached a mature size, the pituitary gland releases another substance called luteinizing hormone (LH). LH carries the message for the "lead follicle"—or biggest follicle—to release its egg. The egg bursts out of the follicle so it can then be picked up by a fallopian tube. The other eggs shrivel and die. (The ovaries release about 400 eggs during the course of a woman's lifetime. Generally the healthiest eggs are released early in life. Although a woman can still become pregnant as she ages, she is much less fertile than she was in her youth.)

• The *fallopian tubes* reach from the uterus to the ovaries. At the end of each tube near the ovary are lush, fingerlike projections called *fimbriae*. When a mature egg is ready to be released, the fimbriae must actively seek out the egg and pick it up from the surface of the ovary. (The egg does not just fall into the tube.) Once the fimbriae have picked up the egg, it is transported by

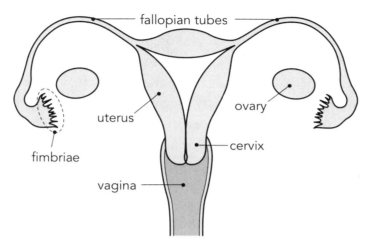

Figure 1.2—*Ovaries and Fallopian Tubes*

little hairlike projections on the surfaces of the cells on the inside of the tube toward the uterus. In the portion of the tube
known as the ampulla, the sperm and egg meet and fertilization takes place.

- The *uterus* is the size and shape of a pear. Its outer wall is a
  thick muscle that is lined on the inside by a narrow mucous
  membrane. The uterus is large enough to hold a quarter tea-
  spoon of liquid, but it can expand to the size of a full-term
  fetus. Early in the menstrual cycle the hormone estrogen
  causes the lining of the uterus to thicken. Later in the cycle,
  the hormone progesterone causes the lining to secrete nourish-
  ing substances to support a fertilized egg that may have implanted itself in the uterine lining.

The Male's Role

It was once assumed that it if a couple was unable to produce a child,
it was the woman who had the fertility problem. That assumption—
though not entirely gone from society—has faded in recent years, and

the male's role is being more closely examined. Male factor infertility is found in approximately 50 percent of infertile couples.

To sire a child, the male must have more going for him than just the ability to ejaculate during intercourse. He must produce a sufficient number of normal, actively moving sperm. Those sperm need an open pathway to pass from the testicles (where they are produced) and out of the body through the penis. The sperm then must be able to travel up through the mucus produced by the woman's cervix, into the uterus, and then through the fallopian tubes to reach the egg. Once in the fallopian tube, the sperm must be able to penetrate and fertilize the egg. Whew!

To impregnate his partner without medical assistance, each part of the male reproductive system must be healthy and in good working order. The parts you should be familiar with are illustrated in figure 1.3 and include the following:

- The *urethra* is a tube that runs from the bladder to the end of the penis. Both urine and semen leave the body through the

---

Male Infertility

According to the definition supplied by the Mayo Clinic, a man is said to be infertile when either of these conditions exist:

1. He produces too few sperm. Even with millions of sperm in each milliliter of seminal fluid, he still may be infertile. About 20 million sperm per milliliter of fluid is considered the lower limit of male fertility.

2. The sperm he produces is abnormal in shape or motility (ability to move) and thus unable to reach or penetrate an egg.[1]

urethra. (Blood fills the cavities along the urethra to make the penis erect while having intercourse.)

- The *scrotum* is the sac hanging behind the penis that holds the two testicles and the epididymis. The *testicles* make sperm and the male hormone, testosterone. The *epididymis* is a long curled tube where the sperm grow and mature.

- The *seminal vesicles* make fluid to help the sperm mature while in the epididymis.

- The *vas deferens* is a tube that carries the sperm from the epididymis to the prostate gland.

- The *prostate gland* makes the fluid that sperm move in.

- *Cowper's glands* put mucous liquid into the urethra right before ejaculation. This liquid helps the sperm move easily through the urethra and out of the body.

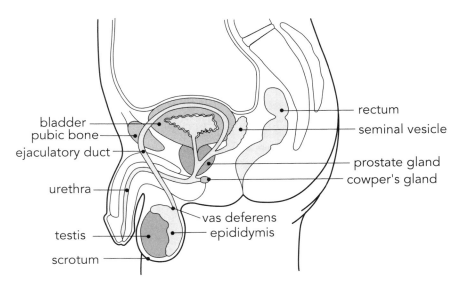

Figure 1.3—*Cross-Section of Male Pelvis*

THE FACTS ABOUT INFERTILITY

There are two kinds of infertility. *Primary infertility* applies to couples who have never had children—they have never been able to conceive after a year of unprotected intercourse or to carry a pregnancy to a live birth.

On the other hand, more than half of the women who are infertile are already moms. Infertility that occurs after a couple has already conceived and delivered a child is called *secondary infertility*. For some women, this inability to conceive again is directly related to the earlier pregnancy and childbirth; a postpartum infection, for example, can cause adhesions in the uterus or fallopian tubes and interfere with future fertility. But in most cases, the reasons for secondary infertility are the same as those that cause primary infertility (as explained later in this chapter). These problems may have developed since the earlier pregnancy, or they may have always been there but have worsened with age.

> ## Sperm Teamwork
>
> It takes sperm teamwork to fertilize an egg. There are protective cells surrounding the egg. Many sperm actively remove these cells to gain access to the egg. Only after these cells have been removed and a path cleared can a single sperm penetrate and fertilize the egg.

The standard definition of infertility also includes women who have repeat miscarriages. (In medical terms, these incidents are referred to as *spontaneous abortions*, but given the lay understanding of abortion as a voluntary termination of pregnancy, the word *miscarriage* will be used in this book.) These women are able to conceive but unable to carry the fetus to a viable age. In the general population, it is not unusual for a woman to miscarry; in fact, chances are one in five that any clinically recognized pregnancy will end in miscarriage.[2] But two, or certainly three, miscarriages without a successful pregnancy in between are reason to suspect an infertility problem.

The medical community is now also aware of cases in which multiple subclinical pregnancies last only days rather than weeks. This subclinical pregnancy is called *biochemical pregnancy* because the only evidence of its existence is a positive blood pregnancy test.

WHEN TO WORRY

It is impossible to say exactly how many months separate the time from when you decide to try to conceive a child and the time you should seek help for infertility. Some people conceive on the first try, but other perfectly healthy and fertile couples do not conceive for several years and then achieve pregnancy without any medical intervention at all. So many individual factors are involved that even the standard "1 year" or "6 months after age 35" suggestions cannot be taken as a rule or a law.

Although it is impossible to predict accurately how long it takes a fertile couple to conceive a child, some generalized statistics can be gleaned from research on the subject. Sherman Silber, M.D., states in his book, *How to Get Pregnant with the New Technology*:

> Modern studies have shown that with the most fertile population of patients (those who eventually went on to raise large families) there was only about a 20 percent chance in any given month of the wife's becoming pregnant. If she was not pregnant after six months, the chance that she would become pregnant in the seventh month was still 20 percent. . . . Each succeeding month the chance for pregnancy is no less in normal women who have not yet conceived than in those who were lucky enough to become pregnant in the very first month.[4]

Dr. Silber goes on to explain that if the conception rate in a large group of normal young women (under the age of 30) trying to achieve

---

Good News About Secondary Infertility

A 1997 study of women receiving fertility treatments found that those who already had children were more likely to give birth again than those who hadn't. The difference was greatest for women under 35 (whose chances were about 7 percent higher) and smallest for those over 40 (for whom the increase was only 2 percent).[3]

Lisa and Paul: Accepting a Single Blessing

Lisa was 28 years old when she and her husband, Paul, decided to start a family. After about a year of trying without success, they began to worry. Lisa had polycystic ovary syndrome (explained on page 23), which caused her menstrual periods to be irregular, so she decided to ask her doctor for some help. As a first step, he prescribed Clomid as a hormone treatment to stimulate the ovary to begin ovulation at the right time. "In the first month on Clomid, I became pregnant, so I'd call that an easy and very successful treatment!" laughs Lisa. A healthy son, whom she and her husband named Jake, was born 9 months later.

During the 2 years after Jake's birth, Lisa took birth control pills to avoid another pregnancy. Then she and Paul decided they'd like to give Jake a brother or sister. Jake is now 4 years old and still does not have a sibling. "I guess it wasn't necessary to be on the pill all that time, but who knew?" says Lisa. "After about 9 months of trying without medication nothing happened, so my doctor again suggested I try Clomid."

Now it's 14 months later, and still no pregnancy. "The last time it worked so quickly that I'm disappointed right now," Lisa says. "We're starting to think, 'What if?' and trying to decide where to go from here if this doesn't work. We have a great little boy, and I think

pregnancy in a given month is 20 percent, about 94 percent will be pregnant within the first year.

The Age-Old Issue

These numbers apply only to "normal young women—under the age of 30." That's because, as we now know, age plays a significant role in determining a female's fertility. A woman is born with a finite number of eggs, which gradually get ovulated or die off as she ages. Older

we could be happy with just the three of us, but I would like Jake to have a brother or sister."

Lisa is finding that the feelings that accompany secondary infertility are very much the same as the ones that go along with primary infertility. "Sometimes," she admits, "I feel like I'm not doing what women are supposed to do. Women have done this without a problem for centuries. Why doesn't my body function like everybody else's? Some days I feel more sensitive about this than others, but my husband has been very supportive, and that's a big help. I think he'd love to have another child in the family, but he says that anytime I want to stop taking the medication and settle back and be happy with what we have is fine with him. I'm just not sure how long we will keep trying and hoping.

"I'm 34 years old now," Lisa adds, "and I know that the efficacy of Clomid decreases after about 6 months, so at some point we'll have to decide to move on. We talk about adoption and foster parenting, and I think these might be options for us. But this is it as far as medical treatments go. I'm not going to get into shots and artificial insemination or any of that. We are a good and strong family as is, and at some point I may have to accept that and be happy with the blessings I have."

eggs, which are less energetic than younger ones, have a harder time making it through the fertilization process. There's no getting around the fact that the older you are, the less fertile you are.

Dr. Silber continues:

For women in their late twenties and early thirties, the probability of conception is somewhat lower, in the range of 10 to 15 percent each month. In such a group only about 70 to 85 percent will achieve pregnancy within the first year. As women get older (in their thirties), the monthly chance of conception is much lower; a failure to get pregnant after a year is likely to mean their monthly chance of natural conception is so low that waiting any longer without treatment would be foolish.[5]

The American Society for Reproductive Medicine (ASRM) agrees. In fact, it financed an ad campaign in 2001 to remind women that time is running out. You might have seen one of the ads on the side of a city bus. The warning "Advancing age decreases your ability to have children" was accompanied by a picture of a baby bottle–shaped hourglass.

> *Older eggs, which are less energetic than younger ones, have a harder time making it through the fertilization process. There's no getting around the fact that the older you are, the less fertile you are.*

Dr. Michael Soules, president of the ASRM, says that a confluence of social factors has created an "epidemic" of women rendered infertile by age.[6] This warning addresses the problem of repeat miscarriages as well. Miscarriage rates jump from 25 percent in the 25 to 30 age bracket to 40 percent in the over-40s.[7]

Although this message is based on medical fact, many women are insulted by it on two fronts: (1) It implies that the woman is solely responsible for infertility (ignoring the various medical reasons that may play a part), and (2) it assumes that having children is something that most women can schedule without considering their marital, financial, or personal state. Although the ads make some feel like the finger of blame is pointing in their face, representatives of the ASRM believe that far too many woman are not aware of the role that age plays in fertility, and these ads are meant to avoid the heartbreak of finding out too late.

Whatever your opinion or life situation, age is a factor you will need to consider when you start to wonder whether you have an infertility problem.

Medical Reasons

The age factor pertains to women without medical reproductive problems. If you are not a "perfectly healthy, normal" couple, the odds of conception and live birth change again. If you have any medical conditions known to interfere with conception or pregnancy, you may not want to wait for nature to take its course. If, for example, you are female and have polycystic ovary syndrome, endometriosis, or pelvic inflammatory disease, after just several months of trying to become pregnant your doctor might suggest a medical intervention. Or, if you're male and know you've had a case of chlamydia that may have done some damage to your reproductive system, why wait to find out?

EVER-GROWING NUMBERS

Gathering correct numbers to define the problem of infertility is not easy or even standardized. Theresa Venet Grant, president of the Inter-National Council on Infertility Information Dissemination (INCIID), tells us, "The numbers are very inaccurate because fertility clinics are required to report to the Centers for Disease Control only the number of couples in their practice who receive some kind of in vitro fertilization procedure." What about those who use other treatment methods? What about those who choose to adopt? And who could possibly know the number of couples who remain childless without seeking medical assistance?

> *Gathering correct numbers to define the problem of infertility is not easy or even standardized.*

Although the numbers may not be totally accurate, the fact is if misery loves company, you should feel great. The ASRM tells us that infertility affects approximately 6.1 million American women and their partners—about 10 percent of the reproductive age population.[8] Figures 1.4 and 1.5 show you visually the one in six couples who are infertile and the 1 in 10 who seek medical help because of infertility.[9] Some believe that in this generation these numbers are becoming an epidemic.

Although the situation has not yet been scientifically documented to the satisfaction of all fertility experts, certainly more couples seem

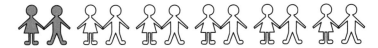

Figure 1.4—*Number of Couples Who Are Infertile*

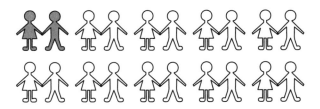

Figure 1.5—*Number of Infertile Couples Who Seek Medical Treatment*

to be experiencing fertility problems than in the past. According to the Family Growth Survey Branch of the National Center for Health statistics, in 1982 (the earliest year for which statistics are available), 12 percent of American women between the ages of 15 and 44 sought infertility services. In 1995, 15.4 percent of women in that group sought help.[10] To handle the growth, the fertility business in the United States has boomed from about 40 in vitro fertilization clinics in 1986 to more than 370 today.

Reasons proposed for this increase are many. Some feel that the sexually promiscuous 1960s passed around sexually transmitted diseases that now, years later, cause both male and female reproductive problems. Others point to our toxic surroundings full of "environmental estrogens" caused by the breakdown of certain pesticides and plastics that are linked to reduced sperm count, endometriosis, and fibroids. The ready availability of legal abortions has caused many scarred fallopian tubes. In addition, the increasing number of women who postpone having children until their 30s or 40s naturally reduces the fertility pool. It's also possible that in 1982 more couples accepted their infertility without seeking medical treatment, unwilling even to think about the brave new world of in vitro fertilization.

HISTORY OF HUMAN FERTILITY STUDIES

In his article, "A History of Human Fertility," James Aiman gives these very interesting facts that make it clear that although infertility has plagued couples since the beginning of humankind, the last 100 years have supplied the greatest advances in our understanding of human reproduction and solutions to the problem.[11]

In about 1200 B.C.E., an early fertility test in ancient Babylonia suggested the following: "To know a woman who will bear from a woman who will not bear: Watermelon pounded and bottled with the milk of a woman who has born a male child; make it into a dose. To be swallowed by the woman. If she vomits, she will bear. If she belches, she will never bear." It was 900 years later when Hippocrates (circa 300 B.C.E.) proposed a more advanced test for fertility: "If a

The Debate over Decreasing Sperm

In 1992, Niels Skakkebaek of the University of Copenhagen, Denmark, and colleagues reported that sperm counts had dropped by about 50 percent worldwide between 1938 and 1991. Their results spawned much scientific study, but experts are still debating whether there really has been a global fall in sperm count or whether the apparent decline is more a reflection of geographical variations. "I don't think we'll ever have an answer to the question of whether sperm counts are falling because designing a study to answer it is exceedingly difficult," says Steward Irvine of the Medical Research Council's Reproductive Biology Unit in Edinburgh, United Kingdom.[12]

Sue and Bob: Young, Healthy, and Infertile

The odds seemed to be in favor of 22-year-old Sue and her 24-year-old husband, Bob. They were both young and very healthy, and neither smoked nor drank. They assumed they would easily conceive a child, but after 4 years of trying unsuccessfully, they are now in the middle of the infertility "journey." "I knew it was time to get a medical opinion," says Sue, "and my husband didn't complain about the idea. I think at that point he'd do anything to shut me up! I was so emotional and upset."

So at the beginning of this year, Sue and Bob both went to visit their family doctor to tell him about their worries. "I really wasn't upset when the doctor used the word *infertility* and referred us to a fertility specialist. We went there knowing something was wrong, and we were hoping for some kind of magic solution. The referral to a reproductive endocrinologist seemed like just what I was hoping for. At that time, I guess I assumed that a specialist could wave a magic wand and something wonderful would happen. It gave me a lot of hope. I was also very glad that our family doctor was quick to decide that our case was beyond what he could handle. I know other infertile couples who have spent years with their family doctors before they get a referral to a specialist, and by that time, they've got the age issue to deal with. I'm really thankful that my doctor knew we needed to see a specialist."

At the first visit to the reproductive endocrinologist, Sue and Bob sat down together and talked with the doctor about their medical and sexual histories. "He really had high hopes for us," Sue recalls. "He didn't find anything in our past that could affect fertility, and he

woman does not conceive, and wishes to ascertain whether she can conceive, having wrapped her in blanket, fumigate below with oil of roses, and if it appear that the nostrils and mouth know that of herself, she is not unfruitful." (This is not as wacky as it seems. Hip-

knew we were young and healthy. Although he was careful not to make us any promises, I felt so relieved and hopeful when he said, 'I think I can really help you.' "

The reproductive endocrinologist immediately referred Bob to a urologist, and Sue and Bob began their fertility workup at the same time. Sue had a couple rounds of blood draws to monitor her hormone levels and a procedure called a *hysterosalpingogram* (a radiographic procedure in which a special dye is injected into the uterus to evaluate the uterus and the fallopian tubes). All test results showed no reason for infertility. Bob was tested for hormone levels and then asked to "donate" more sperm samples than he cares to count. "We live about an hour away from the hospital lab," says Sue, "so my husband had to go to the hospital to give his 'samples.' At first he found this strange, and he felt uneasy. But now he's gotten used to it, and it doesn't seem so odd anymore. He's such a great guy, and he realizes that a lot of men are going through this and it's not such a big deal."

After this series of diagnostic tests, it has been found that Bob has a high number of abnormally shaped sperm that are probably not able to fertilize an egg without some medical assistance. Sue and Bob have now entered the world of fertility acronyms where they are trying treatment procedures such as IUI, IVF, ICSI, and ZIFT (all explained in detail in chapter 3). They still have high hopes and are looking forward to their upcoming first attempt at in vitro fertilization. Like all infertile couples, they keep their fingers crossed and hope that medical science can give them what they most want— their own baby.

pocrates' theory was that if the scent could travel from the vagina to the mouth, the tubes of conception were open and unobstructed.)

During the time of Aristotle (also circa 300 B.C.E.), knowledge of embryonic development was limited. Most believed that the fetus existed in a miniature, fully developed state within the ovaries. Boys came from the right ovary and girls from the left. Others believed that the testes regulated reproduction, and fully developed boys came from the right testis and girls from the left testis.

By 1150, infertility remedies had not advanced greatly. In this time, massages to relevant parts of the anatomy and ingestion of asses' dung were recommended as effective treatment. (See, you do have something to be grateful for—you will not be eating donkey manure as part of any medical treatment!)

As medical science moved into the middle of the first millennium, reproductive knowledge improved little by little. In 1552, Bartolomeo Eustachio advised a husband to insert his finger into his wife's vagina after they had intercourse to push the semen into the cervix. The woman did conceive, and this case may be the first recorded instance of artificial insemination.

The 1600s offered further insights. In 1651, William Harvey contended that the fetus was not preformed, but developed only after the union of a male and female component. By 1668, infertility concoctions had advanced to herbal remedies. Sir Kenelm Digby advised, "An excellent remedy to procure conception consists of the syrups of Mother-wort and Mugwort, Spirit of Clarey, root of English Snake-weed." In 1677, Antonie van Leeuwenhoek used his own invention, the microscope, and was the first to see sperm.

Medical doctors in the 1700s and 1800s began to understand more about the process of conception and were better able to understand why some women were infertile. In 1786, over 100 years after Leeuwenhoek first saw sperm, Lazzarro Spallanzani proved that sperm were essential for conception. John Hunter reported a successful instance of artificial insemination using the husband's sperm. In 1843, Martin Berry observed fertilization in a rabbit, and Oscar Hertwig described the union of the sperm and egg nuclei during the process of fertilization. In 1866, J. Marion Sims successfully inseminated a woman with sperm from a donor. He was also one of the first to time the fertile period of women correctly. In 1871, Karl Sigmund was the first to propose that women menstruated because they failed to conceive.

The wealth of knowledge amassed during the 20th century is especially impressive when viewed in relation to the slow progress previous to this time. The 1900s opened the door of hope and possibility to infertile couples all over the world:

- In 1905, it was suggested that a shift in basal temperature might be related to ovulation. In 1929, scientists in Japan and Germany proved that ovulation ordinarily takes place 12 to 16 days before menstruation. These were both important pieces of the puzzle when trying to determine the best time for conception.

- In the mid-1940s, Max Huhner described the complex interaction between sperm and cervical mucus. This observation is the basis of the postcoital test used extensively today to evaluate infertile couples.

- In 1978, the first "test tube" baby was born in England through in vitro fertilization (IVF—the process in which the eggs from a woman and the sperm from a man are fertilized in a culture dish [in vitro] in an incubator over a 48-hour period, and then the fertilized eggs are implanted in the woman's uterus a few days later).

- In the early 1980s, the U.S. government ordered a complete freeze on any support for medical research on IVF. All research was then financed and supervised through private programs.

- In 1985, Ricardo Asch proposed the process called gamete intrafallopian transfer (GIFT) in which the sperm and unfertilized

> *The wealth of knowledge amassed during the 20th century is especially impressive when viewed in relation to the slow progress previous to this time. The 1900s opened the door of hope and possibility to infertile couples all over the world.*

egg are loaded into a small catheter and placed directly into the woman's fallopian tube where fertilization takes place naturally.

- In the 1990s, fertility research took off at an unprecedented pace. Researchers learned how to stimulate the ovaries to get more eggs, when to give the ovulatory triggering hormone HCG, how to monitor the growing follicle with ultrasound, how to retrieve the eggs without surgery through ultrasound-guided needle aspiration, how to place multiple embryos instead of a single embryo to increase the pregnancy rate, and even how to freeze extra embryos.

The ability to promote fertility in infertile couples continues to make great strides. Many of the latest diagnostic and treatment possibilities are discussed in chapters 2 and 3.

REASONS FOR FEMALE AND MALE INFERTILITY

If you find that you may be infertile, one of your first questions may be "Why me?" You see other men and women having no trouble having babies—even when they don't intend or want to. You want to know "What's the matter with me?" In many cases, the cause of infertility is rooted in an identifiable medical cause, which in many instances is treatable and then fertility can be attained. A variety of these causes for both males and females is discussed in this section; their diagnosis and treatment are explained in later chapters.

> *Although estimates vary, infertility is unexplained in approximately 20 percent of cases.*

Other times, the reason for infertility can't be determined. Although estimates vary, infertility is unexplained in approximately 20 percent of cases.[13] In these cases, some couples opt to try various medical fertility treatments that might increase their chances of conceiving, or they may decide to keep trying the old-fashioned way and investigate other factors that

growing and functioning normally. Certain disorders, such as thyroid disease or diabetes, are also sometimes associated with recurrent pregnancy loss.

Male Factor Infertility

So-called *male factor infertility* is usually caused by a problem with sperm: the number of sperm may be low (viability), the sperm may be abnormally shaped (morphology), or they may move too slowly or sluggishly (motility). The reasons for most sperm problems are unknown. As you can see from table 2, the most common known causes are varicocele, infections, immunological factors, anatomical defects, and hormonal factors.

luck. Statistics indicate that one in five pregnancies spontaneously abort on their own, and I believe Penny's third miscarriage was just one of those." Dave and Penny hope that the next pregnancy will give them the child they long for, but each failed pregnancy brings Penny further into her 30s, and she and Dave know the chances of success diminish with time and age.

"From the outside looking in, it seems like we live a charmed life," admits Dave, "but there is something missing that we want very much. At first you like to think that this kind of thing couldn't happen to you, but here it is. I have to admit this is embarrassing for me, but it's also frustrating. It's hard to see so many neglected and abused children out there when I know we would be very good parents. If Penny's next pregnancy is not successful, adoption may be the next step for us. Right now, it's most important for me and my wife to stick together. Infertility is one of the hardest things a couple can face. It's just not easy."

Table 2. Male Factor Infertility

Varicocele	40%
Unexplained	25%
Infections	20%
Immunological factors	5%
Anatomical defects (other than blocked tube)	5%
Blocked tube	3%
Hormonal factors	2%

Source: Adapted from M. Sara Rosenthal, *The Fertility Sourcebook* (Lowell House, 1998).

Varicocele

If your sperm characteristics are abnormal, it is possible that the source of infertility is a condition called *varicocele*, or varicose veins of the testicles. This condition causes a dilation of the veins and an increased volume of blood in the testicles. Blood retained around the testes leads to an increase in temperature, which can damage sperm and cause low sperm counts and misshaped sperm. Varicoceles may also interfere with testosterone levels.

The role of varicoceles in male infertility is a very controversial topic and always hotly debated among fertility experts. Some researchers and physicians believe that varicoceles are the largest single cause of male infertility, occurring in about 40 percent of infertile men.[18] (However, the incidence of varicocele is found in the majority of all men, fertile and infertile combined.) Others say that many men with varicoceles are able to father children naturally and doubt the condition plays a major role in infertility. Although it's true that most men with varicoceles are able to father children, abundant evidence indicates that the condition is detrimental in some degree to male fertility.

A study by the World Health Organization (WHO) on over 9,000 men showed that varicoceles are commonly accompanied by decreased testicular volume, impaired sperm quality, and a decline in the function of Leydig cells (the cells that make testosterone).[19] This is a particularly common problem for men who are experiencing secondary infertility in which they have already fathered one or more children but cannot father additional children.

Infections

Infections in the reproductive organs can cause reduced sperm production—sometimes temporarily (when the infection is treated with antibiotics before any physical damage occurs), other times permanently. Some infections are caused by various venereal diseases, especially gonorrhea, that can scar the delicate tubes (vas deferens) through which sperm are transported. Tuberculosis or mumps may also invade the reproductive organs and cause physical damage. Viral diseases such as mononucleosis and hepatitis and any other illness that causes a persistent high fever can temporarily but dramatically depress sperm production.

Medical Terms

As you research male infertility (or read your own medical records), you may come across these medical terms that describe the state of your sperm:

Oligospermia: low sperm count

Asthenospermia: slow-moving sperm

Teratospermia: abnormally shaped sperm

Azoospermia: no sperm

Anatomical Problems

Several anatomical abnormalities can make it difficult or impossible for your sperm to do the job. These include retrograde ejaculation, testicle problems, blocked or missing ducts, and abnormal urethral opening.

Retrograde ejaculation. The testes send sperm out of the body through the tube called the urethra. The bladder sends urine out of the body through this same tube. If the bladder neck doesn't completely close during ejaculation, the semen is propelled backward into the bladder instead of continuing down the urethra and out the tip of the penis. When this happens, sperm are then mixed with the urine in the bladder and excreted during urination. (You'll know this is the case if urine passed after ejaculation is milky colored.)

> *Although it's true that most men with varicoceles are able to father children, abundant evidence indicates that the condition is detrimental in some degree to male fertility.*

Testicle problems. Trauma to a testicle, a hernia repair, or bladder surgery can cause the testicle to twist inside the scrotum (a condition called torsion). If left untreated, the testicle shrinks and withers away to the size of a pea, causing infertility. Some males are born with one or both testes still inside the abdomen. This condition is called an undescended testicle or cryptorchidism. Often the testicle descends by itself during infancy without medical intervention, but sometimes surgery is required. An undescended testicle can lead to infertility because sperm cannot be produced in a warm environment, as is found in the abdomen. Sometimes, even after treatment, the sperm count may remain very low. This condition is a risk for the development of testicular cancer and should be medically treated.

Blocked or missing ducts. A variety of congenital defects can cause male infertility. Often the problem is found in missing or defective vas deferens or missing seminal vesicles. (Remember, the seminal vesicles make fluid to help the sperm grow while in the epididymis, and the vas deferens is a tube that carries the sperm from the epididymis to the prostate gland.) Men born to women who took the medication diethylstilbestrol (DES) to prevent miscarriage may experience this problem.

Abnormal urethral opening. You may have been born with a congenital abnormality that places the opening of the urethra on the under or upper side of the tip of the penis. When this is the case, ejaculated sperm are not deposited directly into the cervix. Plastic surgery can construct a new opening at the tip of the penis and close up the old opening.

Hormonal factors. An imbalance of "sex" hormones can cause a number of infertility problems in a male. These pituitary hormones are regulated by a "releasing factor" (called *gonadotropin-releasing hormone* [GnRH]) produced in a part of the brain called the *hypothalamus*. GnRH stimulates the pituitary gland to produce and release the two hormones essential to reproduction: follicle-stimulating hormone (FSH) and luteinizing hormone (LH). In the male, FSH helps stimulate and maintain proper sperm production. LH stimulates and maintains production of the male hormone testosterone. In most cases of male hormonal imbalance, doctors can do much to improve hormonal production and influence fertility. A study reported in the *New England Journal of Medicine* has found that some men who have an acquired case of hypogonadotropic hypogonadism may be successfully treated. This condition is characterized by a deficiency of GnRH. In this study, 10 men who were sexually mature but infertile were found to have hypogonadotropic hypogonadism; fertility was restored in 5 men who received long-term treatment with GnRH.[20] Other treatments involve gonadotropin (FSH/LH) injections or clomiphene citrate to increase sperm production.

Other Possibilities

A number of other reasons may explain why a male is infertile. A few of these include the side effects of testicular cancer treatment, a hypothalamic or pituitary disorder, germ cell dysplasia (the cells that produce sperm are abnormal), and the inability to reverse a vasectomy effectively.

One other factor that often gets little attention in the review of male fertility is age. Although men have been known to "plant their seed" successfully into old age, Susan G. Mikesell, Ph.D., a psychologist in Washington, D.C., who works with infertile couples, says, "Both the count and quality of a man's sperm can decline as he gets older."[21] Her belief is now backed up by a scientific study that says that the further a man is past the age of 24, the longer it takes for him to make his partner pregnant, regardless of her age. The research, published in the European journal, *Human Reproduction*, is the first to provide clear evidence that the age of a man, as well as that of a woman, could be an important factor. The study examined whether men become less fecund as they get older, as opposed to less fertile. (*Fertility* refers to the ability to produce a baby, and *fecundity* to the ability to do so in a certain period of time.)

"It tells us that, to some degree, men as well as women have a biological clock that starts ticking as they get into their 30s," said Dr. Chris Ford of St. Michael's Hospital in Bristol, England, who led the study. "It also indicates that paternal age is another factor to be taken into account when doctors are looking at the prognosis for infertile couples." The research involved 8,500 British couples whose preg-

---

Boxers or Briefs?

Based on a study presented in the *Journal of Urology,* a man's underwear type does not affect his fertility. Despite the common wisdom that briefs raise scrotal temperature and can weaken fertility, this study found no scientific evidence to support the recommendation that men switch to boxers.[22]

nancies were planned and successful. It found that the probability it would take more than a year to conceive nearly doubled to about 15 percent when a man was over 35, from about 8 percent when he was under 25. The chance of a man making a woman pregnant within a year of trying decreased by 3 percent for every year he was over the age of 24.[23] However, some argue that the age of the wife was not controlled for in these studies; therefore, the effect may just be due to the fact that wives of older men tend to be older as well.

COMBINED INFERTILITY

In many cases, the male and the female both contribute to their state of infertility or face factors that can be found in either the male or female. The female may have a mild case of endometriosis, and the male may have a borderline sperm count. The female may have thick cervical mucus; and the male, poor sperm motility. Some sources say that as many as 30 percent of infertility cases are caused by a subfertile condition in both the male and female. This is one more reason many fertility experts insist that the fertility of both the male and female should be tested.

Another condition found in both males and females that can interfere with conception is the presence of antisperm antibodies. (*Antibodies* are protective agents produced by the body's immune system in response to a foreign substance.) In the male, antisperm antibodies attack the sperm and make it difficult for the sperm to make the journey up to the woman's egg. In the female, antibodies attack the sperm, believing them to be foreign invaders. Antibodies to the tail can slow down a sperm. Antibodies to the head are more worrisome and are known to decrease fertilization of the egg. But because couples who have tested

> *Some sources say that as many as 30 percent of infertility cases are caused by a subfertile condition in both the male and female. This is one more reason many fertility experts insist that the fertility of both the male and female should be tested.*

positive for these antibodies still sometimes conceive a child, this is a debatable reason for infertility.[24] If your doctor determines that autoantibodies are the cause of your infertility, it is recommended that you get a second opinion before beginning any kind of medical fertility treatment.

Genetics, too, can influence fertility in both the male and female. Some men have defects in the genes of their Y chromosome, which may affect the development of the system that produces sperm. In one such circumstance, the male may have *Klinefelter's syndrome*, in which he has an extra X chromosome, changing the typical male XY pattern to an XXY pattern. The result is a total lack of sperm (azoospermia).

Some women have a genetic condition known as *Turner's syndrome*, which is the most common genetic defect contributing to female fertility problems. These women have either a missing or a damaged X chromosome (normally, women have two X chromosomes). This condition causes them to be short (generally not growing beyond about 4 feet, 7 inches) and also lack many secondary sexual characteristics such as breasts or pubic hair. They have irregular or nonexistent menstrual cycles and are usually infertile.

Some men and women are born with *Kallmann's syndrome*. This is a condition characterized by infantile sexual development and an inability to smell. Because the pituitary cannot produce LH and FSH hormones, the woman must take hormone supplements to achieve puberty, to maintain secondary sex characteristics, and to achieve fertility.

INFERTILITY OF UNKNOWN CAUSE

Sometimes there's just no explanation for infertility. Your doctor will call this *idiopathic infertility*. All tests are normal, and still a woman does not become pregnant. This scenario, of course, is especially frustrating. If nothing is wrong, there is nothing to treat—a seemingly rather hopeless state. But all is not really hopeless. David Guzick, M.D., of the Department of Obstetrics and Gynecology at the University of Rochester Medical Center in New York, says, "The overall prognosis for pregnancy among couples with unexplained infertility is quite good, especially in younger couples and among those who have been experiencing infertility for 3 years or less."[25]

THE EXPECTED COURSE

If you're like most males and females of reproductive age, in the absence of an obvious medical problem, you probably have never given much thought to your state of fertility. You have assumed you were fertile and would naturally bear children without much ado when you were ready. You probably haven't asked a medical opinion on the necessity of using some form of contraception when you wanted to avoid pregnancy because you assumed it was necessary. And when you stopped using a contraceptive, you were excited about becoming a parent.

It is a very slow process of awareness that brings us to even consider the possibility of infertility. The first month, the second, the third go by with slight disappointment, but not too much concern—after all, it's not unusual for conception to take a while. But then 6 months, and 9 months, and then a whole year goes by— perhaps another year and another. Now what?

> *It is a very slow process of awareness that brings us to even consider the possibility of infertility.*

At that point, it's usually the woman who mentions her concerns to her gynecologist. The gynecologist will examine the history of the case—your age, your partner's age, how long you've been trying to conceive, your general state of reproductive health—and may then decide that it's time to find out whether there is a medical reason you haven't been able to conceive. This doctor may run diagnostic tests him- or herself or may refer you to a reproductive endocrinologist who specializes in the diagnosis and treatment of infertility. (More on this kind of doctor in chapter 2.)

Once the diagnostic testing is completed, your doctor will suggest an assortment of possible treatment options (as explained in chapters 3 and 4). It is up to you to decide how much time, money, and emotional energy you want to invest in treating your infertility. Some couples will try anything no matter how long it takes or how much money it costs, knowing all the time that there is never a guarantee that they will become natural parents. Others will choose not to put themselves through the fertility struggle and opt instead to adopt or remain childless (as discussed in chapter 5). There are no right or wrong choices. You and your partner have to decide together what is best for both of you. This book is written with the hope of giving you the knowledge you need to make that choice.

CHAPTER 2

Diagnosis of Infertility
Getting Some Answers

I F Y O U A N D your partner have "tried everything" and still haven't been able to conceive a baby or carry a pregnancy to term, you are probably ready to begin the process of getting a medical diagnosis. This decision can bring mixed feelings. Of course, you're anxious to find out whether anything is wrong and how it can be fixed, but you may also be worried about what's ahead of you once you take this step.

Veronica A. Ravnikar, M.D., chair of the Department of Ob-Gyn at Saint Barnabas Medical Center in Livingston, New Jersey, says it's vital to know what you're getting into. "It's important to understand what an infertility workup is all about in advance," she warns. "Infertility testing in the male is a little easier because it begins with a sperm analysis, and then you work your way to other tests that are based on those results. But in the female it's a composite of different tests that look for ovulatory function and structural normalcy that have to be done at specific times in the cycle. When you go for your first visit, you may feel overwhelmed when you hear that you'll need one test at this point in your cycle, and another at this date in your cycle, and so on. This can be very confusing.

"It's not like any other testing process you've been through," Dr. Ravnikar continues. "Some of the tests must be done during the day, and they will pull you out of work and your normal activities. You may need to make many visits that are inconvenient and time-consuming. To better understand why this is necessary, you should completely understand the menstrual cycle and the diagnostic process."

This warning isn't meant to scare you out of pursuing infertility testing; it's offered instead as a word of advice that can help you get the most out of a sometimes difficult process. In this case, forewarned is definitely forearmed. According to Dr. Ravnikar, "You should clearly define with your doctor the plan of action. Know exactly what tests will be given, when they will be given, and when all the results will be pulled together. Too often people get lost in the process. They go through some testing and then forget to come back for repeat testing. Then they call and ask for the results and have to hear that they are incomplete and inconclusive. There are so many different appointments that have to be kept at exactly the right time, it does get confusing."

This chapter will give you a look at the diagnostic process that most physicians use so that you'll be better prepared for what's to come and be able to make decisions based on a basic understanding of the procedures, rather than on raw emotion.

FINDING THE RIGHT DOCTOR

Before you jump into fertility testing, it's best to take time to look where you're going. The first step is to carefully choose the physician who will guide you through this process. To begin the infertility workup process, most often the woman sees her gynecologist first, but most professionals in the field of fertility and reproduction believe that management by a trained fertility specialist is vital to successful care. Theresa Venet Grant, president of the InterNational Council on Infertility Information Dissemination (INCIID), feels strongly that the greatest shame of infertility treatment in this country is that women are not referred in a timely fashion to the appropriate special-ist. "If you have been trying to conceive unsuccessfully for 1 year or if you are over 35 and trying for 6 months," says Grant, "you need to see a doctor who specializes exclusively in treating couples with infer-tility problems. If the doctor is also delivering babies, he or she is probably not the right one for you."

If you do decide to go to a fertility specialist, choose this person carefully. Many obstetricians/gynecologists (ob/gyns) and urologists will say that they are well trained to treat someone who is infertile, although in fact they may not be. Mark Perloe, M.D., a fellow of the American College of Obste-tricians and Gynecologists, warns, "Any physician can be listed as a fertility specialist. There is no regulation, licensing, or certification required for advertising this specialty." A listing in the tele-phone yellow pages, certificates on the office wall announcing membership in the American Soci-ety for Reproductive Medicine (ASRM), or com-

> *Most professionals in the field of fertility and reproduction believe that management by a trained fertility specialist is vital to successful care.*

pletion of a short postgraduate course in infertility alone does not qualify one as an infertility specialist. Before you make your first ap-pointment, you should inquire whether the physician is board certi-fied or board eligible in reproductive endocrinology.

To be board certified in reproductive endocrinology, a physician must successfully complete requirements for board certification in obstetrics and gynecology and in addition attend a 2- to 3-year fel-lowship in reproductive endocrinology, pass a written examination on the topic, finish a 2-year practice experience in reproductive en-docrinology, and then pass a 3-hour oral examination. Some doctors have completed all but the oral examination and are still in their prac-tice experience in reproductive endocrinology. These doctors are board eligible in reproductive endocrinology. There are about 500 board-certified reproductive endocrinologists in the United States. Another 800-plus doctors are board eligible.[1]

When looking for a fertility specialist, you'll also need to decide whether you want to go to a doctor in private practice or one associated with a group fertility clinic or academic medical center. Both have their pros and cons, and the decision will be made based on many factors, including practical considerations such as which doctors are on your insurance plan and where they are located geographically.

But as you search, Dr. Perloe advises that you should be wary of the "success rates" posted by many doctors and clinics. "A clinic may report that 25 percent of their patients get pregnant within three cycles," says Dr. Perloe. "So you may assume that you have a one in four chance of pregnancy if you go to them. These could look like pretty good odds to some couples. However, the clinic's statistics do not show that they eliminate more than half of the applicants before attempting any in vitro procedures. So in actual fact only 25 percent of the remaining half of their patients (or really 12.5 percent of all their patients) actually succeed. Don't get me wrong. Many of these clinics are quite reputable and do show impressive results. Just try to be objective when you read or hear about their services and success rates."[2]

Before you make your first appointment, you should inquire whether the physician is board certified or board eligible in reproductive endocrinology.

Don't forget, too, that males need a specialized health care provider. It is unlikely that a man's general practitioner can adequately perform the necessary diagnostic tests, and if this doctor does the tests, he or she will likely refer him to a specialist when the results are in anyway.

Most often men are referred to a urologist, but keep in mind that not all urologists are adequately trained to handle fertility problems. Jean Fourcroy, M.D., Ph.D., from the Uniformed Services University of Health Sciences in Bethesda, Maryland, recommends that all men with suspected fertility problems see an andrologist. Andrology is a specialty within the field of urology that focuses specifically on fertility. Andrologists are the most highly qualified physicians to deal with all aspects of male factor infertility. These doctors have completed a 1- to 2-year program in andrology.

How to Find a Fertility Specialist

You can find a specialist who is board certified in a reproductive specialty in a number of ways:

- Look in the *Directory of Medical Specialists*, published by Who's Who, which is available at most public libraries; it lists all specialists and their training.

- Contact the American Association of Clinical Endocrinologists at www.aace.com or ASRM at www.asrm.org. (See complete contact information in the appendix.)

- To check on a physician's credentials, contact the American Board of Medical Specialties ([847] 491-9091; Web site: www .ama-assn.org), or try the M.D. finder at www.medseek.com.

- You can also contact the organization RESOLVE, a consumer nonprofit organization that provides education, advocacy, and support to those struggling with infertility. It has surveyed many doctors across the nation and has more than 700 physicians who are on the RESOLVE Physician Referral List. By calling or writing the RESOLVE national office (see contact information in the appendix), you can obtain specific data on the physicians regarding their medical training and special expertise and interests.

Questions to Ask the Specialist

When you locate a physician you might like to work with, take time to ask some questions. RESOLVE suggests you start with the following:

- What are their fee structures, payment plans, and insurance coverage?
- Does the doctor or the nurse have a call-in time so that you can ask questions about your case?
- Is the lab and ultrasound office open on weekends and holidays?
- Can procedures (such as inseminations) be done on weekends if needed?
- If it is a group practice, ask whether you will be seeing only one doctor or several doctors in the practice.
- Ask which hospitals the doctor has admitting privileges to.
- If relevant, ask whether the doctor refers to a particular urologist for evaluation of the male.
- Ask whether the doctor does assisted reproductive technologies (IVF, GIFT, or others). If so, are such procedures done there or at a different location?
- Is the doctor a member of the ASRM?[3]

WHERE TO START?

Infertility is not "her" problem or "his" problem. It is a couple problem. So you should start the diagnostic process together. You both need to be examined and evaluated, but it is also important to remember that you both need each other for emotional support.

> *You both need to be examined and evaluated, but it is also important to remember that you both need each other for emotional support.*

Paul R. Gindoff, M.D., professor and director of the Division of Reproductive Endocrinology, Fertility, and IVF at George Washington University Medical Center, believes the emotional aspect of fertility testing should always be considered when a couple begins a fertility workup. "I understand that by the time a couple comes to me as a specialist," he says, "they have probably already been through some kind of evaluation by another doctor and may have already been through some kind of treatment. They may be on clomiphene citrate for over a year and frustrated by the lack of results. Or they may be without treatment and struggling quietly with the tension and anxiety of the situation.

"There is always a lot of emotional fallout and pain involved in infertility," Dr. Gindoff explains. "The diagnostic process you go through only ratchets up the level of tension by making you feel like you're literally under a microscope—checking the quality of your partner's sperm and how well you ovulate, sizing up your masculinity and femininity. When you deal with sex and procreation, it hits on your self-esteem very quickly. The doctor needs to talk about the emotional factors and the stress effects. He or she can't just order some tests and send you on your way. Being forewarned and knowing in advance that this process can be emotionally difficult is the best way to begin."

YOUR MARITAL AND SEXUAL HISTORY

Once you begin a fertility workup, there are no secrets. Don't be shocked or shy when you're asked to describe your marriage and your sexual habits. The doctor really does need to know when, how often, and in what position you have sex.

Together, you will be asked to discuss the frequency and timing of your sex life. The doctor needs to know whether it is frequent enough during times of ovulation to make conception happen. Are you using positions that encourage cervical contact and survival of the semen? Does

> *Don't be shocked or shy when you're asked to describe your marriage and your sexual habits. The doctor really does need to know.*

the female urinate or douche after sex? (Not a good idea.) Do you use lubricants of any kind, such as jellies, oils, or even saliva, that are known to be spermicidal? Could compulsive male masturbation be depleting sperm reserves? Have you ever conceived a child with another partner? What kind of contraceptives have you used?

These questions are not asked to make a judgment on the sexual masculinity or femininity of the partners. They are vital pieces of the infertility puzzle. "I remember one case," recalls Dr. Fourcroy, "in which a couple mentioned that they never had sex at a certain time each month when the woman always had a backache. Well, it turned out that the woman had a condition called Mittleschmerz that gave her back pain during the time of ovulation, so the couple never had sex at the one time each month she could have become pregnant." This piece of information was all Dr. Fourcroy needed to figure out why the couple had not been able to conceive a child. Beware the physician who doesn't ask very personal questions.

THE MALE WORKUP

Historically, infertility has been considered a women's disease. Only within the last 50 years has the importance of the male factor contribution to infertility been recognized. The mistaken notion that infertility is associated with impotence or decreased masculinity may contribute to the male's fear of being tested.

A Serious Problem

"In the overwhelming majority of cases of the 25,000 people who visit our Web site each day, the doctor has never tested the partner for sperm deficiency. We know that infertility is a biological problem for the woman in about 40 percent of the cases and a problem for the man in another 40 percent of cases, yet only the woman is tested! This is a serious problem."

—Theresa Venet Grant, president of the InterNational Council on Infertility Information Dissemination (INCIID) at www.inciid.org

"How can I be infertile," a man might wonder, "when I have no problem having an erection, having sex, and ejaculating?" This response is caused by confusion over the difference between infertility and impotence (complete or partial inability of a man to achieve an erection or ejaculation). "Of course, the desire to have sex, arousal ability, and having an erection are all important to the process," says Dr. Fourcroy, "but being able to have sex is not the same thing as being fertile. Having sex does not guarantee that the sperm are strong or plentiful enough to get to the right place at the right time to fertilize an egg."

After You

It's important for the male (and female, for that matter) to know that the goal of fertility testing is not to point the finger of blame. "It's easy for the male to worry that it is his fault," says Dr. Fourcroy, "but that just makes the whole situation more difficult." Both partners are in this together, and both need to be part of the solution.

Drs. Marc Goldstein and Peter Schlegel at the Cornell Center for Male Reproductive Medicine and Microsurgery believe that the male workup may often hold the key to a couple's infertility problems:

Historically, the approach to the infertile couple has started with an evaluation of the female, primarily because it is usually the female partner who has initiated a workup by consultation with her gynecologist. It makes more sense, however, to start with the male partner, whose initial evaluation may be performed rapidly and noninvasively.

Despite the availability of advanced reproductive technologies, detection of the problem causing male infertility and the institution of directed treatment is possible in most cases. This specific treatment of the "male problem" is often more successful, less expensive, and possibly less invasive than ICSI [intracytoplasmic sperm injection] or other assisted reproduction treatments. In addition, about 1 percent of men who present with the symptom of "infertility" will actually have a

> *The goal of fertility testing is not to point the finger of blame.*

serious medical problem causing the infertility that, if left untreated, may jeopardize the man's health or life.[4]

In the Beginning

Drs. Goldstein and Schlegel have created a very informative Web site at www.maleinfertility.org where they outline the diagnostic process for a male. They say, "The most important part of the evaluation of the infertile male is the history and physical examination. Even in this era of 'high-tech' medicine it has been our experience that in 90 percent of cases an accurate impression is obtained from an initial visit after a thorough history, physical examination, and light microscopic examination of a semen specimen."

> If your doctor is not listening to you, it's time to find another doctor.

Dr. Fourcroy agrees. "It is a truism in medicine," she says, "that over 90 percent of the information you need can be gathered by listening to the patient. The nuances of the sexual activity of a couple have a lot to do with fertility." If your doctor is not listening to you, it's time to find another doctor.

Medical History

The first part of your workup should include a thorough review of your present and past medical history. The doctor will want to know about any acute or chronic illness, disabilities, cancer, use and abuse of any drug, lifestyle factors, occupational and avocational hazards (such as exposure to ionizing radiation, heavy metals, or pesticides), as well as any experience with sexually transmitted diseases or any illness with fever over the last 6 months. He or she will also ask you to recall the approximate age of puberty onset and any postpubescent case of the mumps. Your family history may be relevant if parents or siblings also have experienced fertility problems or if your mother was given the drug diethylstilbestrol (DES) to ward off miscarriage during pregnancy.

According to Dr. Fourcroy, "The evaluation must also include a wide range of factors known to affect fertility in either direct or indirect ways. These include visual changes, headaches, smell and taste abnormalities, or recurrent respiratory infections."

You should also come prepared with a list of current and past medications—over-the-counter, prescribed, and illegal. Many drugs affect the male reproductive system by affecting hormone metabolism, by directly altering the creation of sperm, and by affecting the motility of the mature sperm. In addition, some drugs may affect libido. Dr. Fourcroy tells us, "Even antihypertensive drugs may be the cause of impotence; antidepressants and beta-blockers such as propranolol may decrease libido; cigarette smoking may contribute to vasoconstriction and erectile problems." In addition, drugs of abuse such as alcohol, marijuana, and cocaine are directly associated with infertility problems. Given the many ways drugs can affect male infertility, it's important to give your doctor a complete and accurate list.

> *The doctor will want to know about any acute or chronic illness, disabilities, cancer, use and abuse of any drug, lifestyle factors, occupational and avocational hazards, as well as any experience with sexually transmitted diseases or any illness with fever over the last 6 months.*

Your surgical history is important, too. Don't forget to mention any hernia repair or bladder surgery you may have had. Also talk to your parents and siblings about surgeries you may have had as a child and have now forgotten.

Physical Exam

The fertility specialist will give you a physical exam during which he or she will carefully check for various signs of medical or genetic problems. The doctor may include as part of the exam hormone blood tests, a check for possible varicocele, and a prostate and penile evaluation. Here are some details of what you can expect:

Test for hormone imbalance. The physician will order blood tests to measure the level of hormones (such as FSH and testosterone) that are involved in sperm production.

Varicocele exam. To examine a man for a possible varicocele, the physician will feel the scrotum for what some describe as "a bag of worms." These varicose veins will be most apparent while you are standing and will virtually disappear when you lie down. You may be asked to increase abdominal pressure and make the veins more notable by either coughing or bearing down as if having a bowel movement. As explained in chapter 1, a varicocele can cause low sperm counts and low motility.

Prostate exam. The prostate exam is commonly a part of the fertility workup. Although perhaps unpleasant or embarrassing, many fertility specialists feel it should not be skipped. The digital rectal exam allows the evaluation of possible cysts, enlargement of the seminal vesicle, and obstruction of the ejaculatory ducts.

Genitalia exam. An evaluation of the penis and testicles is a routine part of this physical examination. The penis will be checked for normal site of urethral opening, normal length, and any abnormalities on the glans or shaft. The physician will also look for signs of sexually transmitted diseases. The doctor will check the testicles to find out whether they are soft or hard and symmetrical or asymmetrical. He or she will look for any irregular areas and spots of tenderness that might indicate an infection or any fullness that might indicate obstruction.

Sperm Analysis

In addition to the physical exam, you will be asked to "donate" a sample of your semen for analysis. Dr. Fourcroy explains why: "The assessment of the fertility potential of the sexually mature man resides primarily in examination of the ejaculate because pregnancy of the wife is the only other test of this potential. The male has no other way of knowing if he is ejaculating bullets that are meaningful or blanks, or even if there is any sperm in the ejaculate at all. The only way to know this is to look at the seminal fluid under a microscope. The gold standard of evaluation is the semen analysis, a standard that has been improved in the last decades only by computerized methods."

The Bacteria Link

Dr. Bela Molnar of Hungary knew that the reproductive systems of up to two-thirds of men are infected with anaerobic bacteria (such as *Fusobacterium nucleatum* and *Bacteroids fragilis*), which cause infections that usually go unnoticed. She wondered whether these bacteria could be one factor in some men's fertility problems.

Along with her colleagues, Dr. Molnar collected and analyzed sperm samples from 43 infected men. Normally, sperm will swim in a culture medium for a day or more, but even in the samples with low concentrations of bacteria, only 1 percent of the sperm were still moving after 18 hours. At the highest concentration of bacteria, they all stopped moving after 3 hours. If infertile men have asymptomatic infections, Molnar thinks they should be given broad-spectrum antibiotics for 3 months to eliminate the bacteria before beginning in vitro fertilization.[5]

The ASRM reminds us that the sperm analysis can reveal many things about the sperm:

> General semen examination includes determining the time required for the semen to become liquid, and its volume, consistency, and pH (measure of acidity). Microscopic evaluation of the ejaculate can determine the sperm count, motility (percentage of moving sperm), morphology [normality of shape as illustrated in figure 2.1], agglutination ("clumping") of sperm, and the presence of elements other than sperm, such as white blood cells or bacteria. A normal ejaculate has more than 20 million sperm per milliliter. More than 50 percent of the sperm should be moving forward, and more than 30 percent should have normal shapes.[6]

Once is not enough. "The clinician cannot depend on one analysis," says Dr. Fourcroy. "At least three to six samples are necessary,

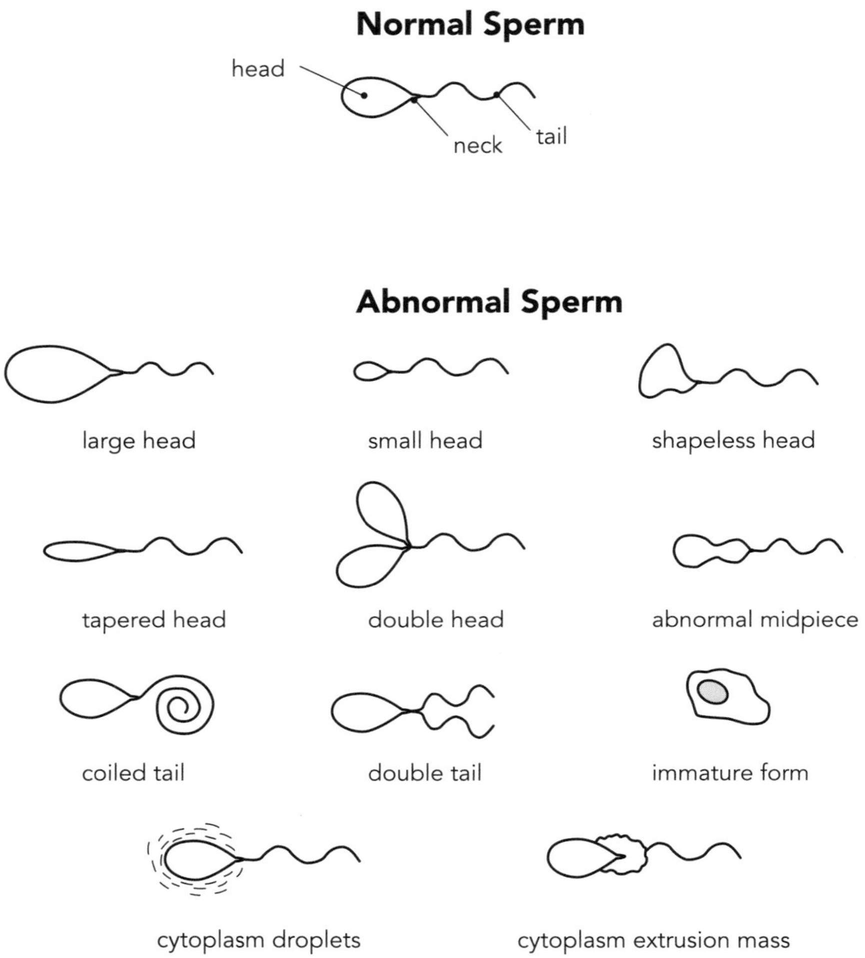

Normal Sperm

head

neck tail

Abnormal Sperm

large head

small head

shapeless head

tapered head

double head

abnormal midpiece

coiled tail

double tail

immature form

cytoplasm droplets

cytoplasm extrusion mass

Figure 2.1—*Sperm Morphology*

each given at least 2 weeks apart, for an appropriate evaluation of the ejaculate sample. An important cause of variability with semen analysis results from changes after illnesses. A common cold with moderate fever of 1 week can result in a documented variation with a drop in sperm concentration 4 weeks postillness, but a return to the baseline concentration at 10 weeks. Both adequate medical history and multiple semen samples separated by several weeks will identify this problem."

A Numbers Game

Dr. Fourcroy believes that the World Health Organization (WHO) standards (shown in table 3) used to evaluate sperm are a statistical game, but she recognizes that they are helpful for comparative analysis. "Based on these standards," she says, "in 1936 it was thought that a male needed 200 million sperm per milliliter to be fertile. In the 1980s this was changed to 80 million. Today the dividing line for 'normal' sperm is cut at 20 million per milliliter. This is the base on which your sperm are evaluated and infertility treatment decisions will be made."

However, Dr. Fourcroy acknowledges that there are always exceptions. "Granted, there are pockets of men who don't follow these rules," she says. "There are some who produce 3 to 5 million sperm

Table 3.   WHO Reference Values of Semen Variables

Volume	2.0 ml or more
pH	7.2 or more
Sperm concentration	20×10^6 spermatozoa per ml or more
Total sperm number	40×10^6 spermatozoa per ejaculate or more
Motility	50% or more motile (grades a + b) or 25% or more with progressive motility (grade a) within 60 minutes of ejaculation
Morphology	Data from assisted reproductive technology programs suggest that as sperm morphology falls below 15% normal forms the fertilization rate in vitro decreases.
Vitality	50% or more live, i.e., excluding dye
White blood cells	Fewer than 1×10^6 per ml
Immunobead test	Fewer than 50% motile spermatozoa with beads bound
MAR test	Fewer than 50% motile spermatozoa with adherent particles

Source: *WHO Laboratory Manual for the Examination of Human Semen and Sperm-Cervical Mucus Interaction,* 4th edition, (Cambridge, MA: Cambridge University, 1999). Reprinted with permission from the World Health Organization.

per milliliter yet routinely get their wives pregnant unassisted. Other men who have had cancer therapy and then rebound after about 2 years, come in for a checkup, and find they have only 1 to 3 million sperm per milliliter, yet they get their wives pregnant on the first try.

There is a lot we don't know, so we can't rely on sperm count numbers alone," she concludes. "Clearly a high quantity of sperm increases the likelihood of pregnancy, but it is not a guarantee of success or failure either way."

Giving Sperm

The semen analysis begins with a process some men find embarrassing, or at least awkward. You'll need to give the clinicians a sample of your semen. The lab will provide instructions to abstain from sex for a certain period of time before the test, and it will give you a small jar to use for the specimen. After masturbating and ejaculating into the jar, either you must take the whole specimen immediately to the lab, or you may be asked to produce a specimen at the lab, where you will use a private room.

> *The process of sperm donation is not physically invasive or overly difficult, but it is not always easy, either.*

The process of sperm donation is not physically invasive or overly difficult, but it is not always easy, either. Writer Peter Landesman describes the experience that many men face:

Worse than being caught at 17 masturbating in bed is being ordered to masturbate at 35 by a strange woman in a lab coat. You go to an anonymous office. They tell you to wash your hands, then they take you to a room. A pile of porn awaits you, to grease the wheels. If you go to an impressive place, they have a video playing out the usual, tired scenarios: Supple Secretary, Eager Interview, Touchy Teacher. Summon your arousal. Imagine rows of closets; imagine the grunts. This is not a lazy, lusty Sunday morning in bed with the wife. This is not the last, tipsy act of an anniversary evening. This is pumping and twitching into a plastic cup. For many of us, this is modern-day fatherhood.[7]

Karen and Rick: Numb from the Numbers

Most couples dealing with male factor infertility have memorized the numbers and percentages relating to sperm count and know exactly how they compare to the norm. When they don't match up, the disappointment and confusion are hard to manage.

When Karen found out that her husband, Rick, had a fertility problem, the mix of emotions was almost too much to bear. "I called my doctor's office yesterday to schedule the postcoital test," she says, "and was informed that we couldn't do it because my husband's sperm count isn't high enough. They said that his semen analysis was 5 million per milliliter, 44 percent motility, with 12 percent morphology. I knew right away that those numbers are not good. My husband will be doing another semen analysis next week so they can double-check the results, but I'm scared that it will be the same.

"Doing the diagnostic testing had brought us new hope. And I feel like it is being torn away. I guess I didn't think it would be him. I thought it would just be me (but something treatable), though my results aren't all in yet. Now I've got so many questions. Is there any hope for my husband's sperm count? Is there anything to increase his count? Is it possible for us to still have a baby? My heart feels like it's broken in a million pieces right now. And the look on my husband's face when I told him the results broke my heart, too."

Optional Sperm Tests

Depending on the results of your sperm analysis, your physician may choose from a number of other tests to gain more information about the sperm's fertilizing ability and to help define specific sperm abnormalities or diseases of the male reproductive system. Your role in supporting these tests is to continue offering your "samples." The ASRM tells us that these tests may include the following:

- Vital staining. Determines numbers of living and dead sperm.

- Antisperm antibodies. Tests for antibodies that bind to sperm and may affect fertility.

- Strict morphology determination. Gives detailed examination of sperm shapes.

- Peroxidase staining. Differentiates white blood cells from immature sperm to assess for possible infection.

- Semen culture. Checks for bacteria that may cause genital infection.

- Hypo-osmotic swelling test. Assesses the sperm membrane for structural integrity.

Jake: No Surprises

The different elements of the male workup add up to a lot of testing that takes its toll on men, who often feel confused about the whole thing. Jake, for example, wanted to "pass" his semen analysis test and was ready to do whatever that would take, but he was worried about conflicting information.

"I have a couple of friends who have gone through this," says Jake. "One of them tells me I shouldn't have sex for at least 5 days before I give my sample. Another says I shouldn't abstain for more than 2 days. My doctor says he's not sure it really matters.

"Well, my wife and I decided to hold off having sex for 4 days before my test, and the results were pretty good. My count was up to a whopping 17,000 with 36 percent motility! That's really noth-

- Biochemical analysis of semen. Measures various chemicals in semen such as fructose (which is absent when there are no seminal vesicles or when the ejaculatory ducts are obstructed).[8]

Additional tests to evaluate sperm function include the following:

- Sperm penetration assay (hamster test). Measures sperm–egg membrane fusion, using hamster eggs and the man's sperm to test the capability of sperm to penetrate the egg during IVF.

- Human zona pellucida binding tests. Measures the sperm's ability to bind to the zona pellucida (outer covering) of the egg. These tests include the hemizona assay, a laboratory test of the ability of sperm to penetrate into a human egg. First the egg is split in half, and then one half is tested against the husband's sperm and the other half against sperm from a fertile man.[9]

ing to brag about, and I have no idea if it has anything to do with how long we abstained, but it was a big improvement over last month's count and enough to make us feel more confident about trying ICSI [intracytoplasmic sperm injection].

"The one thing I've learned through all this is that everyone has an opinion, but there are very few known facts, especially about male factor infertility. I think that's the most frustrating part of this journey—no one can give you a definitive answer about anything. I have known a couple of people with 'morph' problems that wound up getting pregnant naturally. Go figure. Our RE [reproductive endocrinologist] says, 'Nothing surprises me anymore,' and I'm starting to feel the same way."

Further Diagnostic Tests for Men

If your sperm count or quality is in any way abnormal, your doctor might want to do further testing to find out why. He or she might order an ultrasound, a vasography, or a testis biopsy.

Ultrasound. According to Dr. Fourcroy, the ultrasound remains the most valuable, noninvasive, and underused method of evaluating the reproductive tract, including the testis, epididymis, and vas. The ultrasound (also called a sonogram) is a painless technique that uses high-frequency sound waves for creating an image of internal body parts. This method can also be used rectally to evaluate seminal vesicles, ejaculatory ducts, and the prostate.

Vasography. If it is suspected that you may have an obstruction blocking the release of semen, a vasography may be used for further evaluation. This is an x ray of the vas deferens or the ejaculatory duct after they have been injected with contrast dye. Many physicians have replaced this procedure with the less invasive ultrasound.

Testis biopsy. This is a minor surgical procedure performed under appropriate anesthesia or sedation. A small sample of testicular tissue is taken for microscopic examination. The results can be used to help determine the cause of a low or absent sperm count and rule out obstruction.

> *Your partner may feel an increased burden of guilt if you're cleared of "blame." It's important to be sensitive to these feelings.*

The Next Step

If the results of the semen analysis are abnormal, you have several options to pursue, as explained in the next chapter. If, on the other hand, all results are normal, you'll certainly feel a great sense of relief. But the diagnostic process continues with even greater urgency for your partner, who may feel an increased burden of guilt now that you're cleared of "blame." It's important to be sensitive to these feelings. As

The Male Infertility–Cancer Connection

Science has recently come up with another good reason to monitor male infertility medically. Rune Jacobsen and colleagues at the University of Copenhagen in Denmark analyzed the sperm quality of semen samples taken from over 32,000 men in Copenhagen between 1963 and 1995. Sperm count, motility, and shape were assessed. Cancer rates were studied and compared with those expected for the whole population of Denmark to determine levels of risk. Men with poor semen quality overall were between two and three times as likely to develop testicular cancer. Poor sperm quality was also associated with an increased risk of cancers of the abdominal cavity and digestive organs. The researchers concluded that there might be common risk factors for poor sperm quality and testicular cancer, suggesting that these factors may be present in the developing male fetus.[10]

Trish, who is now in this situation, says, "at this point, one wrong word from my husband can just make me explode."

This pain is shared by many women with fertile husbands. In a calmer moment, Trish explains, "Yesterday my husband and I went to his appointment with the urologist. The urologist told us everything looked good with the sperm analysis and ultrasound and that my husband had no fertility problems. His count is at the lowish end of the spectrum, but according to the doctor, it should pose no problems. He was very satisfied with the results and told us it was good news.

"On one hand, I feel better that there is no problem there, but on the other, I sort of wanted an easy explanation for our failure to get pregnant. So now it's my turn, and I'm really worried about what we're going to find. This is so frustrating."

THE FEMALE WORKUP

While your partner is making sperm donations, you, too, can begin the diagnostic process. Your doctor will need to know specifics about your reproductive history. Questions asked will cover sexually transmitted diseases, problems of puberty, fertility in previous relationships, regularity and flow of menses, previously used contraceptives (especially intrauterine devices), use of DES by your mother, eating disorders, endometriosis, diabetes, appendicitis, ovarian cysts, miscarriages, abortions, and abdominal or pelvic procedures.[11] All this information is important to create a complete reproductive medical history.

Physical Exam

You will be given a comprehensive gynecological physical exam. Your doctor will give special attention to the breasts, pelvic area, and genitals. He or she will note the formation and distribution of body fat, abnormal hair patterns, and acne. By pushing against your skin, the doctor will feel your uterus and ovaries, being alert for cysts and polyps. During an internal exam, the doctor will look for irregularities in the size, shape, or position of the cervix and uterus. The doctor may alternately use a sonogram to gain information about the fallopian tubes, uterus, and ovaries.[12]

Diagnostic Tests

After taking your medical and sexual history, the fertility specialist will probably order some diagnostic tests. Before you jump into these sometimes evasive, time-consuming, and expensive tests, take a word of advice from Dr. Gindoff. "The field of infertility diagnostic testing has changed tremendously over the years," he says. "Traditionally, the evaluation of a couple who have not been able to conceive after a year of unprotected intercourse included a variety of tests including the postcoital test, the hysterosalpingogram, a laparoscopy, a hysteroscopy, an endometrial biopsy, and a semen analysis on the male partner. Regardless of the woman's medical history, it was standard to go through a battery of tests before any pronouncement of diagnosis and treatment plan. Now that approach is really out the window. The technology in this field has developed so rapidly, it has replaced a lot of the rudimentary diagnostic tests with a high level of treatment options."

Dr. Gindoff believes that state-of-the-art management uses age and fertility history as the overwhelming determinant as far as what diagnostic tests should be given and what treatment will be recommended. "Because age is driving so much of the infertility work," says Dr. Gindoff, "age now determines the course of treatment. This seems backward, because we naturally think of evaluation first and then treatment, but things have changed. If a woman comes in who is older and we know that she will need fertility drugs along with intrauterine insemination (IUI) or in vitro fertilization (IVF), then we need to put her through very little diagnostic testing before going right to treatment. We would check her FSH level to make sure it is in the normal range, and we would check the partner's sperm count. We could use an x ray called the hysterosalpingogram to assess the uterus and tubal patency if she is going to have IUI with fertility drugs.

> *S*tate-of-the-art management uses age and fertility history as the overwhelming determinant as far as what diagnostic tests should be given and what treatment will be recommended.

"But if IVF is the treatment agreed upon, the sonohysterogram (or hysterosonogram) is done instead of the x ray. This sonogram will evaluate the uterine contour before IVF; this test is much better tolerated than the x ray but doesn't tell much about whether the tubes are open."

This is a new way of looking at age-related infertility. "But," you might wonder, "how can a doctor decide on a treatment if he or she isn't sure my tubes are blocked?" Dr. Gindoff is very practical about this situation: "If a 40-year-old woman has blocked tubes," he says, "it's unlikely that she'll go through the surgery to fix blocked tubes when IVF can bypass that problem. This saves her the time it takes to go through surgery, heal, and try natural conception again. She just doesn't have that kind of time. Even the postcoital test is not necessary if IUI or IVF is the goal. The fertility drugs used along with IUI and IVF will treat the mucus problem if there is one."

If hormone levels are normal and the sperm are acceptable, the only aggressive treatment that can "quickly" get results is IUI or IVF. So, if that's what you're going to do no matter what the reason for the infertility, Dr. Gindoff recommends forgoing extensive and time-consuming testing and moving right to the treatment. (Of course, if the older couple does not want to use IUI or IVF and wants to conceive naturally, then the woman would need the hysterosalpingogram to make sure that her fallopian tubes are open.)

Younger women under 38 have more time to search for treatable causes of infertility, but Dr. Gindoff feels that they, too, should not be subjected to every test in the book without good reason. "If a young woman tells me right in the beginning that she doesn't have menstrual periods on a regular basis (maybe just every 60 to 90 days), I already have my diagnosis: she's not ovulating. I'll check her partner's sperm count and use the hysterosalpingogram to make sure her tubes are open, but that's all. We'll then begin treatment with fertility drugs to regulate her cycle.

> *Women under 30 may be given more extensive testing, because they have time to correct anatomical and medical problems to conceive or carry to term naturally.*

Women under 30 may be given more extensive testing, because they have time to correct anatomical and medical problems to conceive or carry to term naturally. "But," says Dr. Gindoff, "some practitioners follow their nose in a cookbook fashion and give every woman the exact same workup. This just isn't necessary." He feels that if a woman is 43 and is going through every diagnostic test in the book, it is "an absolute waste of her time."

"Any woman over 38 should go directly to a fertility specialist who is a board-certified (or at least fellowship trained) reproductive endocrinologist, not just an ob/gyn who says he or she is a fertility specialist, and begin active treatment," Dr. Gindoff says. "By definition, this person already has a diagnosis: age-related infertility. So why take up so much time testing?"

Female Infertility Tests

The following subsections describe tests that up until about 5 years ago were routinely part of the female infertility workup. Now, like Dr. Gindoff, many fertility experts believe that all these tests are not necessary for all patients. Talk with your doctor before undergoing any testing to be sure that the procedure is needed and that you understand the objective and the expected outcome.

> *Many fertility experts believe that all these tests are not necessary for all people. Talk with your doctor before undergoing any testing.*

Hormone Testing

Hormone levels will be checked carefully through both blood and urine tests. The results of these tests will tell your doctor when you ovulate and whether the right amounts of hormones are present at the right times during your cycle. Because these tests must be timed just right during your cycle, you can save yourself time if you schedule your first consultation during the first week of your cycle. Baseline tests for FSH should be done on day 2, 3, or 4 of your cycle. If your consultation takes place on day 5, you'll have to wait another month for this basic test. Additional tests will be conducted on the day of LH surge (midcycle), and again about 7 days after ovulation to assay progesterone.

Several hormone tests may be given to assess the fertility potential in older women. They can rather accurately predict whether the woman has what is called ovarian reserve failure or, more simply, just not enough good eggs. These tests may be given to help the woman decide whether it is worth the financial and emotional investment, as well as the time, to try to conceive using fertility drugs or assisted reproductive technologies.

According to the ASRM, three common tests are as follows:

Day 3 levels of FSH and estradiol. The determination of blood concentrations of FSH and estradiol levels on menstrual cycle day 3 has been used to estimate fertility potential. Women with elevated levels of FSH and/or estradiol measurements on cycle day 3 have very poor pregnancy rates with both ovulation induction and assisted reproductive technologies such as IVF.

Clomiphene citrate challenge test. To take this test, a woman takes 100 milligrams of clomiphene citrate on menstrual cycle days 5 through 9. Blood levels of FSH are measured on cycle day 3 and again on cycle day 10. Elevated blood levels of FSH on cycle day 3 or cycle day 10 are associated with very low pregnancy rates with both ovulation induction therapy and assisted reproductive technologies.

Response to gonadotropins. Gonadotropins (drugs such as Repronex, Humegon, and Follistim) are concentrated mixtures of FSH and LH (or FSH alone) that are given as injections to stimulate the ovaries to produce multiple eggs in preparation for various fertility therapies. The amount of gonadotropins required to induce egg development rises with increasing chronological age. Women requiring large amounts of gonadotropins to induce egg development generally have lower pregnancy rates with both ovulation induction therapy and assisted reproductive technologies.

> *Ultrasound exams are used to assess the thickness of the endometrium (lining of the uterus), monitor follicle development, and assess the condition of the uterus and ovaries.*

Ultrasound Exams

Ultrasound exams are used to assess the thickness of the endometrium (lining of the uterus), monitor follicle development, and assess the condition of the uterus and ovaries. If the lining is thin, it indicates a hormonal problem. Fibroid tumors and ovarian cysts can often be detected via ultrasound, as well as abnormalities of the shape of the uterus. In some cases, endometriosis can also be detected. Many doctors order a second ultrasound 2 or 3 days after the first. This second ultrasound confirms that the follicle actually did release the egg and can rule out luteinized unruptured follicle (LUF) syndrome—a situation in which eggs ripen but do not release from the follicle. (Some physicians consider this to be a controversial diagnosis.)

Hysterosalpingogram

A hysterosalpingogram (HSG) is a radiographic procedure using x rays to look at the inside of the uterus to check for abnormalities, such as an unusually shaped uterus, tumors, scar tissue, or blockages in the fallopian tubes. The HSG is generally performed in a radiology department. It usually involves placing a speculum into the vagina through which a catheter is positioned in the uterus. Then, radiographic contrast material ("dye") is injected into the uterine cavity. Several x rays of the pelvis are taken.

Although most women report only minor cramping and short-term discomfort during this procedure, some women, especially those who do have blockages, report intense pain. Speak to your doctor about taking a pain medication about 30 minutes prior to the actual procedure.

You should be aware that during this procedure you will be exposed to radiation (as is the case with any x ray), and the contrast

An Unexpected Bonus

Researchers at the University of Texas Southwestern Medical Center in Dallas conducted a study of the hysterosalpingography (HSG) procedure and found surprising results. Almost 30 percent of the 132 women with a history of infertility in the study who were given an HSG conceived within 3 months. The researchers speculate that the dye may exert enough pressure to clear tiny and often undetectable blockages in the fallopian tubes.[13]

material usually contains iodine. If you have an allergy to iodine, a substitute contrast material can be used.

Sonohysterography

Sonohysterography (SHG) is an ultrasound-monitored procedure similar to an HSG. It, too, is mainly used to detect abnormalities of the uterus and sometimes fallopian tubes or tubal blockage.

Sonohysterography can be performed as an office procedure. It usually involves the placement of a speculum into the vagina through which a catheter is positioned in the uterus. Then a saline solution is injected into the uterine cavity, and at the same time, a transvaginal ultrasound is performed.

Some feel the SHG is a safer alternative to the HSG. According to Michael Applebaum, M.D., a board-certified radiologist:

> Sonohysterography, in my opinion, is an excellent procedure for evaluation of the endometrium and tubal patency. It has the added advantages of no radiation exposure, no iodinated contrast injection (which can be associated with increased discomfort and allergic reactions), and the potential for fewer complications. And SHG offers the advantage that ultrasound of the uterus, ovaries, and pelvis can be performed at the same time. Thus, uterine masses and other abnormalities may be discovered which would have been missed during a conventional HSG.[14]

Hysteroscopy

A hysteroscopy allows the doctor to examine the inside of the uterus (as illustrated in figure 2.2). A hysteroscope is a thin tube with a tiny camera on the end. This tube is inserted through the vagina and the cervical canal and placed up in the uterus. Here the doctor can look for a defect in the size or shape of the uterus. "Photos" are taken for future reference.

The hysteroscopy is performed in either the doctor's office or a hospital operating room. You may be given a local or regional anesthetic, which numbs part of your body and keeps you from feeling

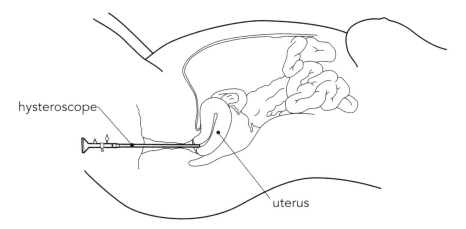

hysteroscope

uterus

Figure 2.2—*Hysteroscopy*

pain, but you remain awake. Or, you may be given a general anesthetic, which puts you to sleep.

Laparoscopy

A laparoscopy is a minor surgical procedure that can help a doctor make a more accurate diagnosis of the cause of your infertility. A laparoscope is a thin metal tube with a tiny light and camera that allows the doctor to look at the organs and tissues in your abdomen. During this procedure, the ovaries and outside of the fallopian tubes and uterus may be visualized and repaired without large abdominal incisions.

This procedure is usually done in a hospital setting. You will be given a general anesthetic, which relaxes your muscles, puts you to sleep, and prevents you from feeling pain. Then your peritoneal cavity, which holds most of your abdominal and pelvic organs, is inflated with carbon dioxide gas. The gas expands the cavity like a balloon and helps the doctor see your organs. As illustrated in figure 2.3, the doctor makes a small cut in or just below the belly button, puts a laparoscope into the abdominal wall, and inserts another tool through a second small cut in the lower abdomen. The scope is guided to look

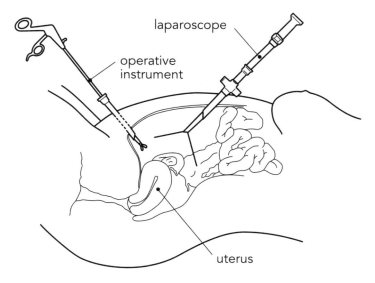

Figure 2.3—*Laparoscopy*

at your pelvic organs and tissues. If the doctor finds a growth that should not be there, the other tool may be used to take a sample of the growth or remove it.[15]

Although laparoscopy is generally acknowledged as the best method for pelvic evaluation, current medical economics and the development of new ultrasound imaging techniques have caused some physicians to reappraise its role in infertility assessments. Stephen Corson, M.D., professor of obstetrics and gynecology at Thomas Jefferson University in Philadelphia, conducted a study of 100 infertile women to find out whether laparoscopy was a necessary part of an infertility workup. All the women in the study lacked a history of prior pelvic surgery, pelvic infection, and signs or symptoms of endometriosis. All had normal pelvic exams and normal hysterosalpingograms (HSGs) and ultrasounds, and their husbands had normal semen parameters. In other words, all had "unexplained" infertility.

"On laparoscopy, however, a total of 68 percent of the women were diagnosed with pelvic pathology that was believed to be of reproductive significance," said Dr. Corson. "The amazing thing was that aside from some Stage I endometriosis, which is what you might expect to find, we had some patients with Stage IV endometriosis, even though they all had normal exams up to this point and no pain." The laparoscopies found tubal problems in 24 women, peritubal adhesive disease in 34, and endometriosis in 43.

Other studies have identified a very small number (5 percent) of abnormalities at laparoscopy that would be attributable to causes of infertility after a normal HSG had been done. Thus, the contemporary role of the laparoscopy has come under debate.

Although the WHO recommends laparoscopy instead of hysteroscopy, Dr. Corson sees value in both. "They're really not competing technologies; they're complementary technologies. If properly performed, the hysteroscopy can be very diagnostic in terms of tubal patency, and it gives information about the inside of the uterus, which the laparoscopy does not."[16]

Postcoital Test

If your doctor thinks that maybe your partner's sperm is having a hard time getting through your cervical mucus to make the trip up to the fallopian tubes, he or she will order the postcoital test (PCT). To perform the test, your doctor will take a swab of your cervical mucus 2 to 12 hours after you have had intercourse. Under microscopic examination, the PCT can detect sperm–mucus interaction problems, the presence of sperm antibodies, and the quality of the cervical mucus.

The timing of the PCT is critical. It is done just before ovulation, when mucus is the most "fertile." PCTs at other times may give false results. This makes it a finicky test for many practitioners to perform.

Falloposcopy

If your doctor feels that your fallopian tubes may be damaged or blocked, he or she may perform a falloposcopy, which allows a visual examination of the inside of the fallopian tube. This procedure involves inserting a tiny flexible catheter through the cervical canal and uterine cavity into the fallopian tube. An even smaller (0.5-millimeter) flexible fiberoptic endoscope is threaded through the catheter into the fallopian tube. The inside of the tube can then be thoroughly examined on a TV monitor via a camera attached to the outer end of the falloposcope.

Abnormalities of the tubes, including obstruction, scar formation, and damage to the inner lining, can be identified. As soon as abnormalities are identified, the doctor can repair the tubes at the same time if that is the best method of treatment. In many cases, the tubes can be repaired through outpatient microsurgical techniques. If tubal damage is too severe to repair surgically, then IVF will be the recommended treatment.

THE DIAGNOSIS OF REPEAT MISCARRIAGES

The occurrence of repeat miscarriages that defines a couple as infertile is in itself a diagnostic process. If you cannot carry a fetus to term on repeated attempts, this is the reason for the medical label of "infertile." Your doctor may then perform further diagnostic tests to determine whether there is a physical reason for the miscarriages.

After taking a detailed medical history, your doctor may order x rays or other procedures (such as a sonohysterography, a hysteroscopy, or an ultrasound) to examine the size, shape, and structure of the uterus. You might remember the story of Dave and Penny described in chapter 1. After two miscarriages, this couple went to a reproductive endocrinologist at Yale Medical Center, and after going through a series of infertility diagnostic tests, found that Penny had a septum in her uterus—a thin wall of tissue that isn't supposed to be there and that aborts a pregnancy. Penny then had surgery to remove the septum and is hoping this will enable her to carry a baby to term.

Blood tests may supply needed information. Your doctor may order a chromosome analysis of both you and your partner; this will evaluate any genetic reasons for the miscarriages. An antiphospholipid antibody blood test may also be ordered; these antibodies (also called the lupus anticoagulant or anticardiolipin antibodies) may cause blood clots, including blood clots in the placenta that prevent the placenta from growing and functioning normally. Your doctor may also order blood tests to check for certain disorders, such as thyroid disease or diabetes, that are sometimes associated with recurrent pregnancy loss.

Your doctor may also perform an endometrial biopsy. This procedure involves scraping a small amount of tissue from the endometrium shortly before menstruation is due. This test is used to determine whether you have a luteal phase defect—a hormonal imbalance that pre-

> Your doctor may order a chromosome analysis of both you and your partner; this will evaluate any genetic reasons for the miscarriages.

vents you from sustaining a pregnancy because not enough progesterone is produced. The biopsy also evaluates whether a condition called chronic endometritis is present. Other hormone blood tests may also be ordered.

A PROCESS OF ELIMINATION

Now 33, Melinda married 5 years ago. She and her husband, James, have been trying to "make a baby" for 2 years with no success. After the first 8 months with no results, Melinda began to wonder whether the chlamydia infection she had at age 18 might be the problem, so she went to her gynecologist to talk about her worries. The doctor suggested a hysterosalpingogram to determine whether the fallopian tubes are healthy and open. The results showed that Melinda's tubes were fine, so she began a series of blood tests that also showed no problems. It seemed that Melinda and James had unexplained infertility.

"After we passed the year mark, when we realized we really might be infertile," remembers Melinda. "We began to get nervous and looked for more information—maybe too much. I began to read everything I could find and thought, 'Maybe I have this; maybe I have that,' and on and on. I began to worry about how everything I've ever done might have made me infertile. I went online and read everything I could find; I got involved in chat rooms talking to all these other women trying to get pregnant and trying all these different approaches. The overwhelming amount of information was making me crazy!"

> *I went online and read everything I could find; I got involved in chat rooms talking to all these other women trying to get pregnant and trying all these different approaches. The overwhelming amount of information was making me crazy!*
>
> —MELINDA

Through this confusing and frightening time, Melinda tried to find answers and comfort from her doctors, but that approach also let her down. "I started with my ob/gyn, and that didn't work at all. Once the tests showed there was 'nothing wrong with me,' she lost interest. Nine times out of 10, I would see the nurse practitioner, and I couldn't get any of my questions answered."

After a year of this, Melinda went to a reproductive endocrinologist who was on the list of approved physicians with her insurance plan. But again, Melinda spent her time with the nurse, rarely the doctor. "I think this happened because I wasn't considered a high-priority case with a definite reproductive problem that could be solved. My husband doesn't have a low sperm count, I'm not over 40, and my tubes aren't blocked. There was really not much to work with."

This new doctor ordered the blood work all over again because he felt the original work had all been drawn at the wrong time of the month, but again everything was fine. The only help he could offer was a prescription for Clomid and then the suggestion that Melinda try superovulation and artificial insemination at least four times or have a laparoscopy and hysteroscopy. "I was so upset," says Melinda, shaking her head. "I had really thought he was going to be able to give me some kind of option that would let us make our baby in our own bed. The whole thing didn't feel right to me, and again, I rarely got to see the doctor. I was just a number in a large pool of women. And although that practice had a success rate that was comparable with other clinics, it just wasn't for me. I realize that they can't always give me the answers I want, but I'd at least like the opportunity to ask the questions."

Melinda then found another doctor 2 hours south of her home who was also on her insurance plan. She admits, "I still see nurses more than the doctor, but everyone is more hands-on and receptive to my questions. And what's more important, they show some compassion. When you're going through this, you feel like hell and really need medical people who acknowledge that." After taking Clomid and Pergonal, working with timed intercourse, and doing an insemination, all without positive result, Melinda and her husband decided to go ahead with the laparoscopy and hysteroscopy.

"Since this was my first surgical experience, I was a bit nervous, but my doctor told me exactly what he was going to do. First, he said I was going to be put out with general anesthesia. Then he would make a small incision within the belly button area and fill the area with gas (this makes it easier for the doctor to maneuver the scope), then basically he would check all around the area for any scarring, endometriosis, fibroids, et cetera. In my case, the doctor found two small polyps on my uterus, and he removed them by making two tiny incisions right above the pubic area. (They later checked these out at the lab and found they were benign.) He performed the hysteroscopy at the same time since I was already under anesthesia. He placed a small catheter with an attached visual tool up the vagina to view the interior of the uterus and tubal openings.

"The entire surgery went without complication and took only about an hour," Melinda says. "The worst part was recovering from the effect of the anesthesia. I was extremely nauseated after awakening. I also experienced pain as the gas they use to fill my cavity dissipated—it required the use of painkillers for 2 days following the surgery. I was back to normal in about a week."

The laparoscopy and hysteroscopy again confirmed that everything was fine. "I know that should be good news, but I really wanted to find out that something was wrong and that it could be fixed," Melinda says. "If everything is fine, what's wrong with us? Sometimes I feel guilty that I can't give my husband a child, and now I'm worried that I'm getting older and this is taking so long. But I'm not going to give up. I knew when we decided to go down the path of fertility treatment that it was a long path and that we had to be steadfast and determined about doing it."

Melinda and James have decided to follow this process through all the way before they give up. "Right now I still have hope. My mother and my sister each took a long time to conceive children, and this gives me a sense of solace. I guess we have choosy eggs! I'm still pretty young and have time. And my doctor said something that really made me feel good. He said that he wants me to try another artificial insemination, and if that doesn't work, he said, 'Let's do an in vitro fertilization and get you pregnant.' Actually, I've been putting off in vitro fertilization because that's my last hope. If it doesn't work, you'll have to scrape me off the side of the road because that'll do me in. But my doctor sounds so confident that it's very heartening to me."

> *I knew when we decided to go down the path of fertility treatment that it was a long path and that we had to be steadfast and determined about doing it.*
>
> —MELINDA

Through this experience with infertility, Melinda says she has learned one very important thing that she would pass on to other infertile couples: "This is a difficult process, and to make it work you have to find a fertility specialist—not a gynecologist—who fits you. You have to trust the people who are going to work with the most intimate part of your life. They have to at least feign concern and compassion for all you're going through. I'm on my third doctor, and now I finally feel good and confident. I think he can really help us make this happen."

Melinda is smack in the middle of today's world of infertility treatment. After enduring rounds of diagnostic testing and coming up without any specific answers, she and her husband moved to the next step. She tried superovulation with hormone drugs and artificial insemination, and she then started the process of in vitro fertilization. Melinda and James now have their fingers crossed as they dream about their future family.

Note: As this book goes to press, Melinda is 6 weeks pregnant after undergoing an IVF procedure called ZIFT, which is explained in chapter 4. She says she is "cautiously optimistic" but undoubtedly thrilled!

Like Melinda and James, many infertile couples go through the regimen of diagnostic tests and then move directly to medical treatments and assisted reproductive technology. But many other couples decide first to try more "natural" methods of enhancing fertility before they begin infertility drugs or other invasive medical treatments. Chapter 3 will give you information about natural fertility strategies that you may want to try.

CHAPTER 3

Basic Fertility Tips and Complementary and Alternative Medicine

WHAT DO YOU do when you find out you have an infertility problem? The answer to that question is a very personal and individual one. Some couples will accept a life without biological children. Other couples will immediately begin to pursue conception through assisted reproductive technologies (as discussed in chapter 4). Still others will take a middle road—one that gives them an active role in improving their state of fertility, but one that is natural, usually noninvasive, and certainly more financially feasible. This chapter takes a look down that middle road at some basic fertility-enhancing tips as well as some of the complementary and alternative therapies that have been used successfully to promote fertility.

FERTILITY 101

The first step many doctors and alternative therapists recommend when beginning the exploration of infertility is menstrual period tracking for the female. This is an especially appropriate, natural method of fertility management if you are still in your 20s (and therefore not rushing to beat the biological clock) and if you realize you're not getting pregnant as soon as you thought you would but are not yet ready to rush into infertility medical treatment. It's also a good place to start if you have "unexplained" infertility and want to give natural conception more time, or if you simply want to conceive naturally without any form of assisted reproductive technology.

Period tracking is a system of charting your menstrual cycle so you know as precisely as possible when you ovulate. If you're just beginning the exploration of infertility, you might wonder, "Why is it so important to know when I'm ovulating?" Knowing this fact is important because ovulation is the process that releases the egg once a month for fertilization. In the healthy female, 10 to 20 eggs will mature in the ovary every month but only one will be released. (Occasionally two will be released and if fertilized will develop into fraternal twins.) This egg will begin its journey down the fallopian tube toward the uterus. It will "live" only for about 24 hours—that's the window of time that healthy sperm have to move up the fallopian tube to penetrate and fertilize the egg. If that doesn't happen in that 24-hour period, you'll have to wait 1 month to try again. That's why knowing when the egg is released is so important if you want to become pregnant.

> *The first step many doctors and alternative therapists recommend when beginning the exploration of infertility is menstrual period tracking for the female.*

Unfortunately, knowing exactly when ovulation occurs is not always so easy. In general, we know that the average menstrual cycle is 28 days long. This means that the "average" woman starts her period on day 1 of her cycle, ovulates on day 14, and after the 28th day will begin to pass menstrual blood again on day 1 of the next cycle. But if your menstrual cycle is 32 days long, you will probably ovulate on day 18. If your cycle is 26 days long, you may ovulate on day 12. This pattern can vary widely, which is why it's important to figure out exactly when *you* ovulate.

Because the egg will live for only 24 hours, you might think that you have to have intercourse on that exact day to conceive a child, but nature gives you a little break here. Sperm can live in the reproductive tract of the woman for about 72 hours. This means that if you have sex on day 11 of your cycle and ovulate on day 14, that sperm still has a chance to fertilize that egg.

The most common methods of period tracking are basal temperature reading and cervical mucus monitoring. The following sections discuss the basics of both approaches.

Basal Body Temperature (BBT) Reading

When ovulation occurs, the increased production of progesterone generates heat in the body,

The released egg will "live" only for about 24 hours—that's the window of time that healthy sperm have to move up the fallopian tube to penetrate and fertilize the egg.

and the body-at-rest temperature rises one-half to one full degree and remains elevated until the end of that cycle. To keep track of when this happens in your cycle, you should purchase a special BBT thermometer and a BBT chart, both available at most pharmacies. Keep this and a BBT chart by your bedside because you need to take your temperature daily before getting out of bed in the morning and record the result on the chart. (The chart may come packaged with the thermometer, or you can make your own, such as the one shown in figure 3.1. As you can see on this sample, you can also chart your menstrual bleeding and days of intercourse for a complete picture of your reproductive patterns.)

The first month of tracking won't help you track your most fertile days because tracking is very useful only in retrospect. The rise in temperature occurs *after* ovulation—when conception is very unlikely or even impossible. Intercourse for the purpose of conception should take place 1 or 2 days before the rise in temperature. (You might notice during this fertile time a slight *drop* in body temperature.) By

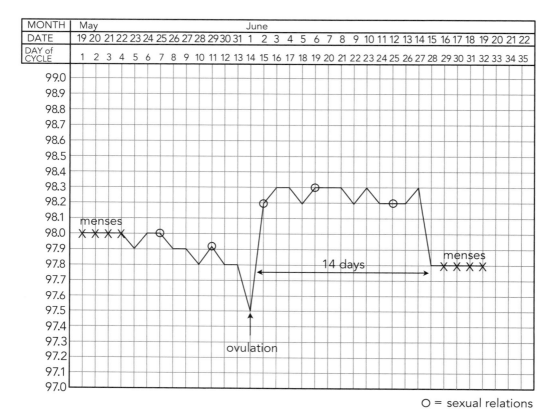

Figure 3.1—*Basal Body Temperature Chart*

keeping a BBT chart for several months, you'll be able to see when the rise occurs and know in the following months which day is your most fertile. If you do not notice any sustained temperature rise during your monthly cycle, you may not be ovulating (even though you get your period). This condition is something your doctor should know about; he or she can prescribe medications to increase the likelihood of successful ovulation.

The BBT is not foolproof. It is influenced by many factors, such as medication, alcohol, degree of physical activity, and illness. So keep track of these things also when you are charting your temperature, and review a period of about 3 months for general patterns. If you do decide to seek conventional or alternative medical treatment, take these charts with you. They will help the doctor or practitioner better work with your individual needs.

Cervical Mucus Monitoring

You have surely already noticed that occasionally you have a discharge from your vagina even when you are not suffering any kind of vaginal infection. Some days the discharge is wet and watery; other days it's thick and sticky. This discharge is giving you important clues about your fertile and infertile days—if you take the time to pay attention.

Inside the cervix are special cells that constantly produce mucus, which, due to changing hormone levels, changes in quantity and quality throughout the menstrual cycle. Low estrogen levels at the beginning and end of the cycle result in scant amounts of sticky or tacky mucus that is cloudy and not stretchy. This mucus has a low pH level and will prevent sperm from traveling up the reproductive tract. As the levels of estrogen rise and ovulation is approached, the mucus becomes more profuse, thinner, wetter, and

> *Intercourse for the purpose of conception should take place 1 or 2 days before the rise in temperature.*

clearer. Then just before ovulation, when the estrogen levels peak, the mucus becomes jellylike and stretchy. (This is called *spinnbarkeit* or *spinn mucus*.)

The quantity and quality of mucus change just before and during ovulation for a good reason. The vaginal area is normally quite acidic, and the cervical mucus is thick, immobilizing sperm and making it impossible for fertilization to occur. But in the few days before ovulation, the mucus changes and provides protection for the sperm, nourishes them, and guides them up into the womb. If you take the time to recognize these changes and combine that information with what you learn by taking your basal body temperature, you'll be better able to predict when you are most fertile.

Evaluating Cervical Mucus

You can easily test the quantity and quality of your cervical mucus by collecting a sample on your fingertips when you sit on the toilet. (Don't use toilet tissue because that absorbs the moisture you need to evaluate.) You do not have to reach your fingers up through the vagina to touch the cervix; the mucus is present right at the mouth of the vagina. It's best to test the mucus several times a day because the changes in hormonal levels can happen rapidly. (First thing in the morning is usually not the best time because after you have lied down all night, the mucus hasn't had time to drain down into the vagina.)

When evaluating cervical mucus, keep track of three things: amount, texture, and color. Record your findings on a calendar, in a notebook, or even on your BBT chart. It will take a few months to see your individual pattern, but one will emerge as you get to know your cycle. You'll see that some days of the cycle leave you almost dry; other days you'll find a thick, sticky substance; and just before you ovulate (the time when you are most fertile), you'll feel the "spinn" mucus (see figure 3.2) that resembles raw egg white and can be stretched about 4 to 6 inches between your thumb and forefinger. It is wet and slippery to the touch and holds together in a jellylike mass.

> **The Water Test**
>
> When testing your cervical mucus, you can distinguish between cervical mucus and vaginal fluids with a simple water test. Dip a sample of the secretion into some water. If it is cervical mucus, it will form a blob and sink, whereas vaginal secretion will dissolve.

Not all women have these exact characteristics in their mucus, but good record keeping will show you the pattern of your mucus discharge on the day before ovulation—the day the sperm can most easily make the journey through the cervical mucus and up the fallopian tube to meet and fertilize the egg.

Ovulation Kits

Many fertility specialists and alternative care practitioners feel it is best to take time to get to know your body and your own menstrual cycle by

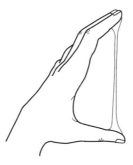

Figure 3.2—*Spinnbarkeit Mucus*

charting BBT and cervical mucus changes, but for some women, over-the-counter ovulation kits are a more convenient way to determine their most fertile days. These kits (which are available in pharmacies) analyze your urine and give a positive result when luteinizing hormone (LH) surges. This surge means that you will ovulate within 12 to 26 hours.

A newly approved test called the TCI ovulation tester measures the amount of saliva in your mouth. You touch a little brush to your mouth and then dab it onto a slide. Looking under the provided handheld microscope at the time of ovulation, you'll see a crystal pattern called *ferning*—it actually looks like a fern plant. The more perfect the pattern, the closer to the exact moment of ovulation.

When either of these tests gives you a "positive," you are in your fertile period and are most likely to conceive if you have sex at that time. Remember, sperm can survive in the female's reproductive tract for 3 days, so if the sperm enter 12 hours before ovulation, they will be ready and waiting for the released egg.

> *Ovulation kits analyze your urine and give a positive result when luteinizing hormone (LH) surges. This surge means that you will ovulate within 12 to 26 hours.*

Timing Is Everything

To maximize your chances of conception, you should have intercourse *before* you anticipate the rise in body temperature that indicates ovulation. Remember: Once ovulation occurs, it is too late for a sperm to

A Bit of Folklore

It's a well-known "remedy" passed from chat room to chat room: Take cold medicine to help you get pregnant. Any truth in this claim? Although there are no scientific studies to back it up, in theory, some doctors agree it might be helpful because the active ingredient in many cough preparations, guaifenesin, softens and thins mucus. Philip McNamee, M.D., president of the Society for Assisted Reproductive Technology in Birmingham, Alabama, says, "Guaifenesin could thin the cervical mucus in a woman whose cervical mucus is thick, allowing sperm to penetrate more easily."[1]

fertilize the egg. The mucus thickens to block the sperm, and the entrance to the cervix grows firmer and closes tightly to prevent sperm from entering. Time intercourse for every other day for 2 to 4 days in this fertile period. Intercourse every other day is recommended over every other hour because ejaculating too often can lower the sperm count. In one ejaculation from a fertile man, more than 20 million sperm are released—this is plenty to do the job until the next group arrives 48 hours later.

Beware of Vaginal Lubricants and Douching

If you use vaginal lubricants, your cure for infertility may be quite simple: Stop using them! According to a 1996 study, commercial vaginal lubricants inhibited sperm motility by 60 to 100 percent.[2] This finding is especially important to know if your partner's sperm is weak in number or function. Petroleum jelly, plain glycerin, and even saliva can act as spermicide and kill sperm. So if you want to get pregnant, give up the lubricants (and even oral sex before vaginal sex). If a lubricant is required for your comfort, try egg whites; they have no known negative effect on sperm and work quite well.

Douching, too, can interfere with the normal reproductive process, so if you douche to clean your vagina, stop. Douching can reduce your state of fertility by disrupting the natural environment: It can change the pH level of the vagina, possibly damaging or destroying sperm. It also can deteriorate the quality of the cervical mucus. Evidence indicates that douching increases the likelihood of an ectopic pregnancy as well. Vaginas are self-cleaning and are best left alone.

If you use vaginal lubricants, your cure for infertility may be quite simple: Stop using them!

LIFESTYLE CHANGES FOR IMPROVED FERTILITY

The fertility tips suggested in this chapter are the basics that all couples should know, but as Clara and José discovered (see sidebar), they will not work for everyone. They will not help the truly infertile female or male who has a biological reason for being unable to conceive or carry to term. In some of these cases, the root of infertility can be found in lifestyle factors that alter the healthy functioning of the reproductive system.

Many of your daily lifestyle habits may be affecting your state of fertility. Changing these habits may be all that's needed to improve your chances of conceiving naturally and having a full-term pregnancy or, if you choose, of successfully completing some method of assisted reproductive technology. This section will help you take a look at the roles of nutrition, environmental toxins, smoking, caffeine, alcohol, medications and illicit drugs, excessive weight loss or gain, rising body heat, and exercise.

Nutrition

Both the inability to conceive and repeat miscarriages may be resolved through a change in diet. Sound incredible? Not if you consider that we already know that diet is a major player in the way the body handles the risk factors for physical diseases and conditions such

Clara and José: Every Trick in the Book

Clara and her husband, José, married at age 33. "We wanted to start our family the day we got married," laughs Clara. "My plan was to get pregnant on our honeymoon." But that didn't happen. In the 5 years since their wedding, Clara and José have "tried everything," Clara says. "First I tracked my periods for 6 months and found that my cycle was 30 to 33 days. Then I wanted to figure out when I was ovulating. Everybody thinks we all ovulate on day 14 of the cycle, but that's not really true. I had to find out in my cycle when the timing would be just right for me. I started taking my temperature every morning before I got out of bed, I tested my cervical mucus all month long, and I bought ovulation kits. I needed to take time to find out more about my own body." To the point of obsession, Clara kept a notebook filled with all the everyday facts of her monthly cycle. She used timed intercourse to coincide with her "fertile" days and had sex only every other day to maximize her husband's sperm count.

This focus on procreation helped Clara learn more about her reproductive cycle, but it also had its downside. Eventually it turned

as stroke, heart attack, cancer, diabetes, autoimmune diseases, and on and on. Why is it remarkable, then, that nutrition should influence the state of one's fertility? Long-term, extensive research studies out of major universities have not yet been conducted to "prove" this relationship between diet and fertility. But the logic behind the connection is sound, and the following recommended diet changes are certainly not harmful. Improving your overall diet will at best improve your state of fertility and at worst reduce your risk of life-threatening diseases. You have nothing to lose.

Peter Degnan, M.D., of Exeter Hospital's Equinox Integrated (East-West) Medicine Center in New Hampshire, agrees. "It is clearly

sex into a chore. "This can really kill your sex life," she admits. "There's no spontaneity anymore. It's more like, 'Hurry up; I'm ovulating today.' Or, 'No, not today; hold on till tomorrow.' This isn't about you and him and lovemaking anymore; this is about trying to make a baby."

For months, then years, Clara and José had sex on a timed schedule, doing everything they could to make the most of it. "We tried different positions," says Clara. "One doctor told us to forget the missionary position and try to enter from the back. Another told me to be on top because my uterus is tipped back. I even laid with my head hanging off the bed trying to get gravity to work with us. (I had a friend who said she did it standing on her head, but that was just more than I could do!) And then I would lie in bed for half an hour after sex with my legs propped up. I'm telling you, we tried everything."

It's been a long 5 years for Clara and José. They are now just about ready to move on. "I still hope that I'll get pregnant and have a biological child," Clara says, "but we're now looking into adoption. To be honest, it's actually a relief to stop trying so hard to conceive."

well known that women who do not take in adequate nourishment have reduced fertility due to the body hindering the release of the egg for ovulation. A general review of basic body needs for calories and the proper composition of foods is very important as a first step in evaluating fertility." Dr. Degnan doesn't recommend any particular foods to increase fertility because there is no scientific backing for such claims and also because couples can make themselves crazy trying to eat only the "right" food at the "right" time. "I recommend wholesome, nutritious foods from whole grains with an emphasis on fruits and vegetables," he says. "I encourage the use of organic foods to reduce the potential for ingesting pesticides and toxins through the food chain. I also think its best to use meat products that have been raised on feed that hasn't had antibiotics added to it."

Dr. Degnan believes that a balanced diet of wholesome foods should supply all the nutrients needed for optimum health. Therefore, there is no need to load up on supplements, which in some cases when overdone can create an unhealthy state. The exception is folic acid. "For women who have repeat early miscarriages based on a neurologic developmental problem," says Dr. Degnan, "folic acid may have some role in allowing a healthy pregnancy to progress to full term." Folic acid is found in leafy greens, whole grains, wheat germ, and soy. If you do conceive, ask your doctor about folic acid supplements to ensure healthy neurological development of the fetus.

> *Improving your overall diet will at best improve your state of fertility and at worst reduce your risk of life-threatening diseases. You have nothing to lose.*

Brian Clement, the internationally renowned director of West Palm Beach, Florida's, Hippocrates Health Institute and author of *Living Foods for Optimum Health*, has seen in many of his clients how diet can influence fertility. To help your body deal with the onslaught of harmful substances you eat each day that aggravate the optimal health needed to support fertility, Clement makes the following recommendations:

1. Switch to an organic-based diet. The pesticides, fungicides, and herbicides, along with the toxic effects of estrogens and biogenetically engineered foods, wreck havoc on the body.
2. Reduce, if not eliminate, the amount of animal fat you take in.
3. Increase the amount of healthy liquids you consume each day: switch to purified water, fresh juices, decaffeinated drinks, and herbal teas.
4. Eliminate alcohol.
5. Eliminate caffeine and nicotine; they gunk up the system with waste products and interfere with the healthy functioning of all body systems.

6. Reduce, if not eliminate, processed foods; they are filled with things like white sugar, preservatives, and many other toxic chemicals.

7. Be aware that part of your daily "diet" is also what you inhale in your environment. Buy nontoxic paints (now readily available in many name-brand varieties). Use woolen area rugs rather than wall-to-wall polyester formaldehyde carpeting. Do not buy clothes that need to be dry-cleaned. Make sure air circulates in your environment: Always keep a window at least cracked in the office and at home. Open your car window just a bit even when it's cold to counter the carbon monoxide continually coming into the car.

> Your goal in using diet as a therapy for fertility is to feed your body only foods that will nourish and support optimum health.

Your goal in using diet as a therapy for fertility is to feed your body only foods that will nourish and support optimum health. The Food Guide Pyramid in figure 3.3 will give you an idea of how you can improve your daily diet. You'll see that this nutritional guideline from the U.S. Department of Agriculture advocates a diet heavy in grains, fruits, and vegetables, with decreasing amounts of milk, yogurt, cheese, meats, nuts, fats, and sweets. Following these basics will help you give your body what it craves to be strong and healthy and eliminate the foods and substances that overburden it with waste and debris.

Environmental Toxins

The air you breathe, the water you drink, the foods you eat, and the chemicals you clean, paint, and renovate with may be the cause of your reproductive problems. Some of the primary culprits have been identified and their effect on fertility documented, but with several thousand commercial chemicals being introduced each year, it is a

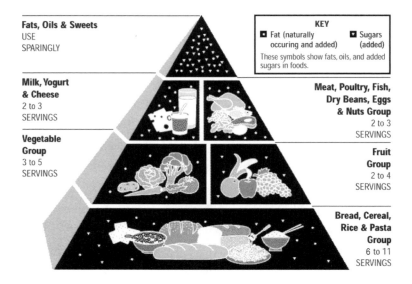

Figure 3.3—*The Food Guide Pyramid*

Source: Centers for Disease Control and Prevention

monumental task to pinpoint each one that can affect human reproduction. That's why it's best as a general rule to avoid any chemical products and toxins.

Environmental toxins can and do affect both male and female fertility. Many toxic substances have their greatest effect on cells that are in the process of growing and dividing. That's why the testicles, which make new sperm every day, are so prone to damage. In fact, the declining fertility rates among males are often attributed to the rise in environmental toxins.

The effect of environmental toxins on the reproductive health of females is most notable in women who miscarry. According to Dr. Gary Berger in *The Couple's Guide to Fertility*, substances having the potential to cause early miscarriage include ethylene oxide, used in the chemical sterilization of surgical instruments; vinyl chloride, used in the plastics industry; chemical solvents used in manufacturing industries; nitrous oxide exposure among anesthetists, operating room doctors and nurses, veterinarians, dentists, and dental assistants; and metallic compounds of manganese, arsenic, and nickel. An increased likelihood of repeat miscarriage is also found in women whose male partners are chronically exposed to lead, the pesticide dibromo-chloropropane (DBCP), vinyl chloride, and anesthetic gases.[3]

Occupational exposure to textile dyes, lead, mercury, and cadmium has also been associated with female infertility.[4] Of course, women who work with these substances are at high risk, but just because you don't work with dyes or metals doesn't mean you *aren't* affected by them. Lead can come from water pipes, flaking paint, or traffic exhaust fumes. Mercury is found in fish caught in contaminated rivers or coastal waters and in dental fillings. Cadmium exposure comes from active or passive cigarette smoking. Other toxins to avoid include copper, sometimes found in water pipes, and aluminum, found in aluminum foil, antacids, cookware, and antiperspirant sprays.

> ## A Video Connection?
> Clusters of miscarriages have been noticed among women who work with video display terminals (VDTs). It is not clear whether VDTs are the direct cause, but caution is called for. If you work with computers, use a protective screen that absorbs radiation, and take frequent breaks away from the monitor.

There are many toxins that both males and females should avoid. Some include pesticides, paint and paint strippers, dry rot or woodworm treatments, glues, and chemicals such as solvents. Even household cleaning agents such as oven cleaners, mold treatments, and ammonia-based products have been shown to have negative effects on the health of sperm and ova.[5] Obviously, this isn't the best time to begin a home renovation or cleaning project. If you must, be sure to protect your skin from exposure, and wear a mask to avoid inhaling more fumes than necessary.

If you have concerns about any environmental toxins you may be exposed to, find out the facts. The following hotlines can help you determine whether your fertility has been compromised and what you can do about it:

Environmental Protection Agency
Safe Drinking Water Hotline
Phone: (800) 426-4791

*E*ven household clean-
ing agents such as
oven cleaners, mold treatments, and ammonia-
based products have been
shown to have negative
effects on the health of
sperm and ova.

**National Coalition Against the Misuse of
Pesticides** (also called Beyond Pesticides) and
National Network to Prevent Birth Defects
Phone: (202) 543-5450

**National Pesticides Telecommunications
Network**
Phone: (800) 858-7378

**National Institute for Occupational Safety
and Health (NIOSH)**
Phone: (800) 356-4674

Smoking

You already know that smoking can cause cancer, cardiovascular disease, and rapid aging. But do you also know it is a primary factor in
both female and male infertility? Now you have one more very strong
reason to give it up.

The case against smoking for females is a strong one. According to
Howard D. McClamrock, M.D., associate professor of obstetrics, gynecology, and reproductive sciences at the University of Maryland
School of Medicine, "Studies have shown that tobacco use can decrease the supply of eggs within the ovaries, even in young women."[6] A
study presented in *Family Planning Perspectives* found that "increased
smoking of cigarettes by women is directly related to the difficulty in
conceiving." It goes on to note that the proportion of women who are
subfertile rises with the number of cigarettes smoked daily.[7]

Men don't get off easy on the smoking issue, either. Research has
shown that 16 cigarettes a day can decrease sperm count and motility,
increase the number of abnormal sperm, and make it less likely that

the sperm will fertilize an egg.[8] Continued smoking can lead to further sexual problems as well. Randolph Smoak Jr., M.D., a surgeon from Orangeburg, South Carolina, noted this relationship in a piece he wrote for the *American Medical News.* He stated that the onset of impotence is related to the duration of smoking:

> Once a man has smoked for more than 10 years, he has an increasing likelihood of impotence based on tobacco use alone. I've often operated on male smokers who have had blockage of the main artery right below the navel, which closed their pelvic vessels. I'm sure it's no surprise that almost 100 percent of them were impotent. We know that erectile dysfunction certainly can occur when the blood vessels that supply the region are constricted.[9]

For your general health as well as your state of fertility, today is a good day to give up smoking.

Caffeine

Caffeine is suspected of having several effects on the reproductive process, including a possible impairment of or delay in conception. This effect was noticed in a large European study of infertility risk factors. A randomly selected sample of 3,187 women aged 25 to 44 years from Denmark, Germany, Italy, Poland, and Spain reported on the time of unprotected sex before their first and most recent planned pregnancies. They also answered questions about their consumption of caffeinated beverages. (In all countries coffee was the principal source of caffeine.) The study found that a significantly greater number of women who consumed more than 500 milligrams of caffeine per day (approximately four cups of coffee) took more than 9.5 months to become pregnant compared to those who drank less.[10]

> Caffeine is suspected of having several effects on the reproductive process, including a possible impairment of or delay in conception.

Caffeine is also known to have a generally negative effect on overall health, so it's a good idea to give it up during this time when you want your body to be exceptionally healthy.

Alcohol

Many believe that drinking alcohol—even in moderation—can affect the fertility of both women and men. In her book, *Getting Pregnant Naturally*, Winifred Conkling says:

> In women, alcohol affects the liver's ability to clear hormonal debris, disrupting hormone levels and interfering with egg production. While the amount of alcohol required to alter brain chemistry and hormone levels varies from woman to woman, evidence suggests that even moderate drinking can contribute to infertility. A 1994 study involving women who used alcohol moderately (one drink or less per day) found a strong correlation between drinking and ovulatory dysfunction and endometriosis.[11]

> *There is no doubt that long-term alcohol use can lead to impotence, poor sperm quality, and further fertility complications due to liver damage.*

The male must also be careful to limit alcohol use to maintain maximum fertility. There is no doubt that long-term alcohol use can lead to impotence, poor sperm quality, and further fertility complications due to liver damage. Provided the liver has not been severely damaged, fertility problems caused by alcohol use may reverse when the alcohol intake is stopped.[12]

Medication and Illicit Drugs

Everything you put into your body has an effect on your overall health and often your fertility—this includes medications and illicit drugs. If you are taking any over-the-counter or prescription medications, be sure to talk to your doctor about their possible effects on fertility. Conkling writes, "A number of drugs can interfere with fertility, including certain antibiotics, antiseizure drugs, antidepressive drugs, antihypertensive drugs, cortisone and corticosteroids, and anti-ulcer drugs. Women who are trying to get pregnant should choose aspirin or acetaminophen instead of ibuprofen, a drug that may disrupt ovulation and implantation of the fertilized egg in the uterus."[13]

An example of a widely prescribed medication that has been linked to infertility is the hypertension drug nifedipine. This calcium channel blocker is sold under many brand names, including Procardia and Adalat. Its infertility effect appears to be restricted to males and is caused by nifedipine's ability to block calcium influx into sperm. At the annual meeting of the American Society for Reproductive Medicine and the Canadian Fertility and Andrology Society, Dr. Susan Benoff of the New York University School of Medicine explained that these drugs alter the cholesterol content of the membrane. Sperm overloaded with cholesterol becomes nonfunctional. The infertility effect is reversible when the drug is withdrawn (making it a candidate for a potential male contraceptive).[14] The direct effect on fertility of most medications is unknown; if you don't absolutely have to take them, don't.

Many illicit drugs are used because they affect the central nervous system and create an altered sense of being. Unfortunately, they also affect the brain's output of both male and female hormones that control the production of reproductive hormones. Changes in concentrations of the pituitary hormones LH, FSH, and prolactin can result in reduced libido, sexual dysfunction, and infertility. Drugs with these effects include amphetamines, anesthetics, cocaine, barbiturates, benzodiazepine tranquilizers, "angel dust," heroin, and marijuana.[15]

Excessive Weight Loss or Gain

Being significantly under or over your ideal weight can affect the level of fertility in both males and females. The ASRM tells us that low weight can lead to a decrease in an important hormonal message that the brain sends to the ovaries in women and testes in men. This hormone, gonadotropin-releasing hormone (GnRH), is produced in the part of the brain called the *hypothalamus*. This release of GnRH leads to the release of the hormonal messengers LH and FSH by the pituitary gland. LH and FSH are critical for the development of eggs in the ovaries and sperm in the testes.

The degree to which weight loss affects fertility will vary. In mild cases the ovaries may still produce and release eggs, but the lining of the uterus may not be ready to receive a fertilized egg because of inadequate ovarian hormone production. In more severe cases, ovulation does not occur, and menstrual cycles are irregular or absent. In men, low weight may lead to decreased sperm function or sperm count.

Being significantly under or over your ideal weight can affect the level of fertility in both males and females.

The ASRM notes that being overweight can also affect fertility by influencing the same hormonal signals to the ovaries or testes. In addition, increased weight can increase insulin levels in women, which may cause the ovaries to overproduce male hormones and stop releasing eggs.[16]

Weight extremes also influence the probable success of assisted reproduction treatments. In one recent study, over 3,500 Australian women who received assisted reproduction treatment between 1987 and 1998 were divided into five groups according to their weight: underweight, moderate, overweight, obese, and very obese. The fertility of the moderate group was almost 60 percent higher than that of the very obese group, and the fertility of the underweight group was also significantly lower than that of the moderate group.[17]

Some of the hormonal imbalances caused by excess weight loss or gain can be controlled through fertility medications such as clomiphene or gonadotropins. But the natural and healthy way to beat this problem and assure a healthier and more successful pregnancy is to address the weight problem before conception.

Rising Body Heat

You've probably already heard that to protect fertility, the male should wear boxer shorts. According to most fertility experts, this claim may or may not be so, but there is some logic to the theory behind the advice.

The testicles hang outside the body in the scrotum for a reason. This is nature's way of keeping the testis cooler than body temperature. It seems that sperm production is best when the testis is a degree or two lower than 98.6 degrees. For this reason, it makes sense to keep the testis from overheating. (Did you know that in Japan hot baths have been used as a method of male contraception?)[18]

There's no harm and nothing to lose by men wearing loose-fitting pants, avoiding hot baths and saunas, dispensing with Lycra shorts during workouts, and keeping their legs uncrossed when sitting. Marc Goldstein, M.D., director of the Center for Male Reproductive Medicine and Microsurgery at New York Hospital, Cornell Medical Center, has found that there is a 2-degree difference between sitting at your desk with your legs crossed and standing outside naked. "Man," he says, "was created to stand up in the woods naked."[19]

Cut the Commute!

Men who drive more than two consecutive hours per day may be at increased risk for male infertility, according to a recent report from French researchers. Results from a study of nine healthy men show that scrotal temperatures were 1.7 to 2.2 degrees Celsius higher after driving for 2 hours than after walking. These findings, say the researchers, could help explain why men whose occupation requires them to drive for long periods take longer to conceive than men who don't drive for a living.[20]

The Good and the Bad of Exercise

Exercise is good for improved fertility, but it can also be bad—it's a matter of degree. Because exercise is an important factor in total body health (which is directly related to one's state of fertility), it is smart to exercise if you are experiencing infertility. Exercise will promote good circulation to all body parts, including the reproductive system. It will reduce the stress of daily life that is aggravated by the stress of being infertile, which compounds the fertility problem. The stress-reducing benefits of exercise occur because exercise pushes the brain to release chemicals such as adrenaline, serotonin, and norepinephrine that can boost mood and relieve tension and depression. Exercise will also promote better sleep, which allows the body restorative time it needs to repair and rejuvenate. And it can help knock off calories for slow, steady weight loss. All of these benefits promote optimum health, which is necessary for improved fertility.

> *Exercise will promote good circulation to all body parts, including the reproductive system.*

However, excessive exercise is known to decrease the state of fertility. Too much exercise can interrupt the normal flow of hormones from the woman's hypothalamus and pituitary. These abnormal hormone levels can interfere with ovulation, menstrual cycles, and therefore fertility. An example of this would be the infrequent or absent menstrual cycles sometimes seen in women who run 15 to 20 miles a week.

Dr. Degnan also cautions women who exercise only moderately to be careful about exercise that raises the internal body temperature. "Exercising to the point where you end up perspiring can work against conception and full-term pregnancy. Walking, swimming, and easy cycling are all good for you, but it's best to avoid working to the maximum aerobic level."

Because of the many similarities in the hypothalamus-pituitary hormone system of men and women, there also may be similarities in the male response to excessive exercise. Dr. Berger tells us that prolonged periods of intense exercise can interfere with a man's rhythmic release of GnRH from the hypothalamus and, subsequently, the release of pituitary hormones LH and FSH, just as in women. For a man, the result can be reduced testosterone levels and lower sperm count.[21]

Exercise can also be harmful to male fertility if it heats up the testicles or involves the use of steroids. As previously mentioned, sperm production can be influenced if the temperature in the testes rises. While you are trying to improve your state of fertility, you might avoid bicycle riding, jogging, or any other exercise in which the testicles are tightly confined, rubbed, or heated and see whether there is any difference in your sperm count.

> *It is well known that the use of anabolic steroids, sometimes used as performance enhancers, can cause long-term male infertility.*

Steroids, unlike exercise, are not a controversial issue. It is well known that the use of anabolic steroids, sometimes used as performance enhancers, can cause long-term male infertility. These steroids are essentially pure testosterone derivatives, which cause an increase in testosterone levels. When the pituitary and hypothalamus glands (which control hormone releases in the body) see a rise in testosterone, they stop producing natural testosterone. As a result, the testes actually shrink in size, and the user's natural testosterone levels dramatically drop. The result can affect the user many years later, even after he stops taking the drugs.

All these lifestyle factors may be having a direct effect on your overall health—and your level of fertility. If you're having trouble conceiving or carrying a child to term, it's a wise idea to get your body in top physical shape so all systems can support the reproductive process. In many cases, complementary and alternative medicine can help you do this.

COMPLEMENTARY AND ALTERNATIVE MEDICINE

Because conventional medicine doesn't have all the answers, many people with infertility problems turn to complementary and alternative medicine (CAM). No one type of CAM has risen above the others as the "cure" for infertility, but many kinds have brought couples to a successful full-term pregnancy. Some CAM therapies commonly used by people with infertility problems are discussed in this section. They add to your list of treatment options that give you some control over how you manage your reproductive health. In this chapter, you'll find a discussion of holistic medicine, natural hormone balancing, acupuncture and traditional Chinese medicine, homeopathy, herbs, physical therapy, and naturopathic medicine.

*B*oth scientific study and anecdotal evidence show that each of these therapies has helped some couples overcome infertility.

Both scientific study and anecdotal evidence show that each of these therapies has helped some couples overcome infertility. This is not an all-inclusive list, however; other therapies are also available that you might want to try. Those discussed in this chapter will give you a place to start.

Holistic Medicine

John Pan, M.D., has been an ob/gyn for 27 years and is also the founder and director of the Center for Integrated Medicine at The George Washington University Medical Center in Washington, D.C. He and his coworkers do not focus their work only on the reproductive systems of infertile couples but rather on the health of the whole person. "We believe that when a person's overall health improves, so do the pregnancy rates," says Dr. Pan.

"There is a model for our work at the University of Surrey in Britain called the Foresight Program that has established a 6-month preconception program in which the emphasis is on detoxifying the body of environmental toxins and attaining overall superior health," Dr. Pan explains. "About 87 percent of their couples have infertility problems. Of that group, those who complete the program have been able to achieve a 90 percent pregnancy rate with no pregnancy loss."

Dr. Pan was so impressed by these numbers that he wanted to try something similar through the Center for Integrated Medicine. His program has expanded on the British program by adding other body-strengthening elements such as nutrition, stress management, acupuncture, and herbs to maximize the couple's health before conception.

"We have a 2-month evaluation period," says Dr. Pan, "during which we conduct medical and genetic workups as well as holistic assessments of both the male and female. Then we enter a 4-month treatment period when we correct any health imbalances through a combination of conventional and alternative medicine.

"Certainly, if a man or woman has a mechanical problem that requires conventional medical attention, he or she is given that, but we have found that many infertile couples, especially those with so-called unexplained infertility, improve their chances of conceiving and carrying to term a healthy child by improving the state of their overall health."

Dr. Pan feels that it is not a waste of precious time to spend 6 months building total health, even for infertile couples in their 30s and 40s. "Even if the woman does not successfully become pregnant and eventually moves on to in vitro fertilization," he says, "her chances of a successful IVF increase dramatically because her overall health is in an optimum state."

We have found that many infertile couples, especially those with so-called unexplained infertility, improve their chances of conceiving and carrying to term a healthy child by improving the state of their overall health.

—JOHN PAN, M.D.

Natural Hormone Balancing

From a holistic point of view, infertility is a breakdown of multiple systems, rather than just the reproductive organs. When a couple is diagnosed as having infertility caused by a hormonal dysfunction, the first line of treatment in conventional medical practices is often the use of fertility drugs such as Clomid, Pergonal, or Follistim to over-stimulate the ovaries. In alternative medical practices, however, the practitioner will first look for the cause of the dysfunction in hopes of rectifying the root of the problem. This can help bring about a natural conception or improve a couple's chances of a successful round with assisted reproductive technology.

Rebecca Wynsome, N.D., is a naturopathic and licensed primary care physician in the state of Washington, where her practice focuses on infertility and women's health care needs. When looking specifically at hormonal dysfunction, Dr. Wynsome will always begin her hormone examination with functional lab tests that check the metabolic activity of the body. Salivary tests in particular check hormonal levels.

"When a woman spits into a new test tube every third day for a month," says Dr. Wynsome, "a compiled graph gives me a complete picture of what her estrogen and progesterone levels look like every day over the course of that month. This is very critical. Without this information, I can't really judge her ovarian reserve accurately. I get much more information from this test than a conventional doctor can get from the standard hormone blood tests taken only a few times during a cycle."

With these results in hand, Dr. Wynsome will check three total-body aspects of hormonal production and function: the creation of hormones, multiple organ systems interaction, and the breakdown and metabolism of hormones.

The Creation of Hormones

Did you know cholesterol levels can cause hormone dysfunction? It's true. Cholesterol lays the groundwork for the production of all hormones. Low cholesterol levels (approximately levels under 170) can't perform this function, so a hormonal imbalance occurs. "Many women that I see (especially vegan or vegetarian women)," says Dr. Wynsome, "need to boost their intake of cholesterol to aid in the conception of a child or to carry to term."

Multiple Organ Systems Interaction

All body systems should be in optimal health to support the process of reproduction. After all, self-survival is a higher priority than reproduction. The body organs tied directly to hormonal balance include the adrenal gland, the hypothalamus and pituitary gland in the brain, and the thyroid gland (as well as the liver and bowel, as explained later). Dr. Wynsome examines the function of each of these to make sure they are supporting proper hormone production and use.

The adrenal gland plays a part in fertility of both males and females. It is the hidden key that unlocks a lot of fertility problems. Dr. Wynsome will again administer a salivary test; this one checks the levels of two hormones that the adrenal gland makes: DHEA and cortisol. "If your ovarian reserve is low *and* your adrenal reserve is low," cautions Dr. Wynsome, "you have much less of a chance of conceiving a child—even if you juice up the ovaries by stimulating them with fertility drugs. Understanding the state of your adrenal gland is very important to understanding the state of your fertility."

The hypothalamus and pituitary gland in the brain are also a focus of natural hormonal balancing. This is where sex hormone production begins. The hypothalamus receives input from the pituitary gland that regulates the release of LH and FSH. From the pituitary, LH and FSH pass

> *The adrenal gland plays a part in fertility of both males and females. It is the hidden key that unlocks a lot of fertility problems.*

through the bloodstream to reach the primary sex organs of the female (the ovaries) and the male (the testes). These sex organs then release the secondary sex hormones: predominant in males is testosterone; and in females, estrogen and progesterone. (Because there is crossover in the synthesis of testosterone, estrogen, and progesterone, small amounts of each hormone exist in both males and females.) Conventional medicine often focuses on where the sperm meets the egg (which is helpful), but Dr. Wynsome prefers, when appropriate, to work at the root of the problem in the brain and get all systems working together.

In some women, thyroid function is subclinically low, which can interfere with hormone production and fertility. This condition won't show up in a blood test, and a conventional doctor might say your thyroid function is in the normal range. "I might look at that," says Dr. Wynsome, "and say, 'It's not clinically diseased, but according to this saliva test, it's not optimal, and we need to get this body system working to enhance the chances of conception.'"

The Breakdown and Metabolism of Hormones

A healthy liver and gastrointestinal tract are necessary to keep balanced hormone levels running through the system. The liver and the bowel break down, metabolize, and eliminate estrogen as new stores are constantly created during each menstrual cycle (or are added during fertility drug treatments). When the liver is functioning optimally, the "old" hormones are effectively removed, and the pituitary and hypothalamus in the brain are signaled to produce more. But if the liver function is weak, the "used" hormones remain in the system. This buildup of hormones throws off the hormonal balance required to support the reproductive system. The health of the liver and gastrointestinal tract, along with the other body systems, thus needs to be addressed before hormonal balance can be expected.

> *When the liver is functioning optimally, the "old" hormones are effectively removed, and the pituitary and hypothalamus in the brain are signaled to produce more.*

Natural Hormone Supplementation

After this kind of body system examination, a holistic medical practitioner will treat the body systems that may be weak and affecting fertility. The remedy may be in the natural therapies discussed later in this chapter, such as acupuncture, homeopathy, or herbs. In many cases, this treatment may restore fertility and allow a couple to conceive naturally, or it will improve reproductive health to a point that will make assisted reproductive technology successful.

In some cases, however, even after the whole-body system is ready to support the reproductive process, the hormone levels remain unbalanced for a variety of reasons. This is often the case, for example, when chronic stress interferes with hormone production. Too much stress will drain the adrenal glands and thus deplete their levels of hormones. When this occurs, the ovarian progesterone is shunted to aid the adrenal glands and thus is not available for ovarian reproduction support. In this circumstance, Dr. Wynsome may prescribe natural hormone therapy that may include progesterone, DHEA, cortisol, and/or estrogen in a carefully regulated and timed ratio.

> *Too much stress will drain the adrenal glands and thus deplete their levels of hormones.*

Natural hormones are compounded hormones made in a lab that are bioidentical to the body's natural hormones. For example, to produce a natural progesterone, the active ingredients are extracted from soy and yams, and they are changed to produce a progesterone that is identical to what is found in the body.

The natural hormones Dr. Wynsome uses are generally administered in pill or suppository form. "Depending on the results of a woman's saliva test," says Dr. Wynsome, "I might give her bi-est (a natural double estrogen) on days 4 through 10 of her cycle to push the body to produce an estrogen peak at that time. Then I might use oral micronized progesterone after that on days 12 through 28. It all depends on the very individual hormone needs of each person, which I can see in the month-long hormone graph from the saliva test. I much prefer natural hormones over the fertility drugs used in conventional medicine when possible."

Most alternative practitioners agree with Dr. Wynsome. Because these natural hormones are more like the hormones the body naturally makes, they have several advantages over the popular fertility drugs:

- They work on the female's body at physiological levels.
- They have fewer side effects.
- The body processes them more effectively.
- Women feel better while on them.

Because natural hormones are more like the hormones the body naturally makes, they have several advantages over the popular fertility drugs.

Natural hormones are available to all physicians through compounding pharmacies that make them. They are not often used, however, because drug companies cannot own a natural substance and therefore cannot profit from their sale; therefore, they do not mass-produce or advertise them—but they are available and are used by many complementary and alternative physicians.

Acupuncture and Traditional Chinese Medicine

Acupuncture is a major Oriental healing art that involves the use of fine needles inserted at specific points on the body. This therapy originated in China thousands of years ago and is based on the theory that an essential life energy called *qi* (pronounced "chee") flows through the body along invisible channels called *meridians*. When the flow of qi is blocked or out of balance, illness or pain results. It is believed that stimulation of specific points along the meridians can correct the flow of qi to restore or optimize health.

Hannah Bradford, M.Ac., of the Center for Integrative Medicine at George Washington University Medical Center in Washington, D.C., uses acupuncture to restore qi to infertile women. "I feel that because acupuncture is so low risk and relatively low cost," says Bradford, "it is appropriate to try acupuncture before you try something else for any presentation of infertility. The options in the medical system are so daunting and the success rate numbers are so low, that this is definitely worth trying, especially for those on the less medically se-

No Longer Voodoo

Miles Belgrade, M.D., a neurologist and acupuncturist from Minneapolis, Minnesota, says, "Acupuncture should no longer be considered in the category of snake oil or voodoo. Unlike many other alternative medicines, acupuncture does have a scientific foundation. It's a foundation that is consistent with the Western scientific thinking."[22]

vere end of the infertility spectrum and for those with unexplained infertility."

The blocks of qi that affect conception and pregnancy are many. An acupuncturist will look for these blocks by feeling the body pulses and meridians. He or she will then likely do a treatment on the "conception vessel" meridian that goes down the front of the body's torso. Other treatments can be added depending on the individual needs of each person. "It's important to consider the whole person," says Bradford. "Constitutional weaknesses are treated with acupuncture, and, in addition, disruptions in energy resulting from overwork, stress, and other lifestyle effects are addressed."

Bradford says that the acupuncture meridians not only regulate the flow of qi but also contain a sort of communication system that, when stimulated, can remind the body how to do something it has forgotten how to do. "In the infertile female, for example," says Bradford, "acupuncture can remind her system how to ovulate correctly. In fact, this is where I find acupuncture most successful. Many studies support the use of acupuncture for ovulatory problems." Bradford notes that acupuncture is also used to improve the blood flow to the ovaries and uterus. This nourishes the reproductive system and makes it more capable of producing and nurturing eggs. Acupuncture can also help the woman who suffers repeat miscarriages by improving the health of the lining of the uterus where the egg implants and develops.

"Acupuncture," says Bradford, "can also stimulate brain function to regulate hormone release and improve overall reproductive health."

Mengda Shu is a practitioner of traditional Chinese medicine (TCM) at the Center for Integrative Medicine at George Washington University Medical Center. Dr. Shu also uses acupuncture to treat many infertile women—both those trying to conceive naturally and those already involved in assisted reproductive technologies. She says, "I have seen acupuncture improve the success rate of women trying insemination or in vitro fertilization." Dr. Shu has found acupuncture to be especially helpful to women who have already experienced failed cycles. If, for example, a woman who is taking fertility drugs still does not produce enough quality eggs to proceed with IVF, Dr. Shu will use acupuncture and Chinese herbs to restore the hormonal balance and reproductive health necessary to have a successful IVF procedure.

> *Acupuncture and Chinese herbs can restore the hormonal balance and reproductive health necessary to have a successful IVF procedure.*

Dr. Shu also believes that acupuncture and herbs can improve the chances of successful transfer and implantation of a fertilized egg. "IVF is going to be more successful," she says, "when there is an abundant flow of energy to the womb."

In addition, Dr. Shu uses acupuncture to treat male infertility caused by low sperm count or poor sperm morphology. "In the male," she says, "infertility can be caused by a kidney deficiency. By stimulating the meridian that restores the circulation of qi and blood flow to the kidney, many weaknesses in sperm production can be corrected."

Dr. Shu's beliefs are supported further by Daoshing Ni, L.Ac., D.O.M., Ph.D., president of the Yo San University of Traditional Chinese Medicine in Santa Monica, California. In a paper he presented to the Pacific Coast Reproductive Society, Dr. Ni emphasizes that TCM can be used alone or in conjunction with assisted reproductive technology (ART) and fertility drugs:

> The following are some of the preliminary results our clinic has seen.
> We have found increased follicular development with some patients

in an ART cycle with combination of TCM and fertility drugs, especially in ones that were labeled as "poor responders." This can be seen in either an increased production of eggs in GIFT/IVF or increased fertilization rate in IVF. Patients who have thin endometrial lining during the usage of clomiphene citrate have found TCM helpful in reducing the thinning of the lining. We also have found some patients who have stopped ART due to symptoms of premature menopause as well as elevated FSH levels have "bounced" back with utilization of TCM. Most women with irregular menstruation or dysmenorrhea have found TCM to be helpful in managing symptoms

Acupuncture can also help the woman who suffers repeat miscarriages by improving the health of the lining of the uterus where the egg implants and develops.

as well as regulating the menstrual cycle. In male subfertility conditions, we have found some cases of improved semen analysis with the use of TCM for more than three months.[23]

A Story of Acupuncture and Determination

Traditional Chinese medicine has helped many couples struggling with infertility achieve their dream of having a birth child. Dr. Shu's impressive history of turning infertile couples into happy parents has made true believers of her patients. Rosamunda is one woman who believes that if it were not for Dr. Shu and her own determination to be actively involved in her reproductive health, her son would never have been born.

"We started trying to have a baby when I was 31 years old," remembers Rosamunda. "After a year without success, my husband and I both went for infertility testing and were told that my husband has a genetic problem that causes poor sperm quality in the male and miscarriages in the male's partner." This was a double whammy for this couple because even if Rosamunda's husband could contribute enough good sperm to result in pregnancy, there was a good chance that she would miscarry.

They went to a second doctor who immediately recommended in vitro fertilization. "I decided I'd rather try artificial insemination first," says Rosamunda. "Cost was a factor, and I also felt very uncomfortable for some reason about IVF. Unfortunately, three inseminations did not work, and one additional cycle was canceled."

Rosamunda and her husband then went to another state for another opinion. Here she was told that due to her own high FSH levels (indicating an ovulatory problem), she was not eligible for their infertility program. "This doctor tells me that based on that one score, I am perimenopausal and that there is no hope for me whatsoever in IVF, even though eight previous scores had been very low, making me, at that time, a great candidate for IVF," says Rosamunda, shaking her head. "He told me that he had done a study of 1,200 women in my condition and that in that group, only 20 conceived, and 12 of those miscarried. He was convinced that I had no chance of having a successful IVF. I questioned this research because it was several years old in a field that is so rapidly evolving. But the doctor was adamant and told me coldly that I should adopt." Rosamunda and her husband later learned a hard lesson about their rejection. "We discovered," she confides, "that many clinics with high success rates are that way only because they take no risk whatsoever with difficult cases."

Traditional Chinese medicine has helped many couples struggling with infertility achieve their dream of having a birth child.

With their hearts broken, Rosamunda and her husband went back to their home-state doctor and began IVF as he had originally recommended. "This doctor worked at a university hospital and was interested in helping couples with difficult cases like ours. He dismissed the other doctor's research and was still optimistic that IVF would work for us."

Rosamunda eventually moved on to another local clinic that had a "shared risk" program. In this program, the couple pays a flat fee (i.e., $20,000) for several IVF cycles and is guaranteed a delivery or else receives a prorated refund. Rosamunda's first cycle was canceled because she did not respond to the fertility drugs. Because she did not ovulate, this attempt did not count as one of her IVF procedures. At that point, the clinic wanted to cancel her out of the program entirely to cut its losses while it was ahead, but Rosamunda was determined to make this work, so she insisted that the clinic hold up its end of the bargain. "We had been accepted into the program after a battery of tests that indicated our chances of success were high. After just one failed cycle that provided the clinic with new information that they felt indicated that my probability of success was now low, they tried to shirk their responsibility in sharing the risk."

The second and third tries were also canceled even though the drug dosages were increased. "Then in the middle of my fourth cycle (which was not going well)," Rosamunda says, "I was reading a book about infertility, and I came across one line that said something about the positive effect of acupuncture. I frantically began looking for an acupuncturist, and that's when I found Dr. Shu."

Rosamunda and Dr. Shu agreed that it would be better to wait out this cycle, use acupuncture for 3 months, and then try IVF again. But because the cycle she was currently in might count as one of her three tries if she should ovulate, Rosamunda decided to begin acupuncture immediately and see whether it had any effect right away. "My medical doctor made it clear that he didn't think acupuncture was going to do anything for me and recommended again that I cancel the cycle. But after just two acupuncture treatments given every other day, I started ovulating and went from zero eggs to seven eggs. After a total of four treatments, I went in for my egg retrieval. Of the seven eggs, four were retrieved. Of those four, only one survived after intracyto-plasmic sperm injection.

"There were a lot of people in that clinic who were really irritated with me for pushing the system and having only one embryo to transfer," Rosamunda says, "but that one is my son today. I'm convinced that we beat the odds because I did what I thought was best for me and not what doctors said I should do."

There's a funny footnote to this story: The day Rosamunda went to the hospital to deliver her baby, the cab driver told her husband that after failing at infertility treatments, his wife's doctor had recently recommended that she try acupuncture. That doctor was the same man who discouraged Rosamunda from trying acupuncture 9 months earlier. "Apparently, we've turned him into a believer!" she laughs.

Acupuncture Basics

Everyone who considers using acupuncture wants to know, "Does it hurt?" The American Academy of Medical Acupuncture says that people experience medical acupuncture needling differently, but most people feel only minimal sensation as the needles are inserted; some feel nothing at all. No pain is felt once the needles are properly in place. Because acupuncture needles are very thin and solid and their points are smooth, as opposed to hollow needles with cutting edges, like hypodermic needles, insertion through the skin is not as painful as injections or blood sampling.[24]

> *People experience medical acupuncture needling differently, but most people feel only minimal sensation as the needles are inserted; some feel nothing at all.*

The number of treatments needed differs from person to person. Bradford feels that positive results should be seen within the first 6 months. If the woman does not become pregnant within that time, then further acupuncture sessions are unlikely to help.

Acupuncture is generally safe, but as with any therapy, you should be cautious. Judith Horstman, author of *The Arthritis Foundation's Guide to Alternative Therapies*, offers the following advice if you decide to use acupuncture:

- Get a diagnosis from a medical doctor before undergoing acupuncture to make sure you don't have a condition requiring prompt medical attention.

- Don't stop your medications without consulting your doctor. Acupuncture works with, not instead of, conventional medicine.

- Tell the acupuncturist about all health conditions, and list all medications (including herbs and nonsteroidal anti-inflammatory drugs that could cause you to bleed, for example).

Finding an Acupuncturist

To find a list of accredited acupuncturists, contact the following organizations:

National Certification Commission for Acupuncture and Oriental Medicine
Phone: (703) 548-9004
E-mail: info@nccaom.org
Web site: www.nccaom.org

American Academy of Medical Acupuncture
This organization offers a list of medical doctors and osteopathic physicians.
Phone: (800) 521-2262
Web site: www.medicalacupuncture.org

- Be sure the acupuncturist uses sterilized or disposable needles.

- Don't take muscle relaxants, tranquilizers, or painkillers right before acupuncture because acupuncture can intensify the effects of these drugs.

- Tell the practitioner right away if you experience pain. Acupuncture shouldn't hurt after the initial sting of the needle's insertion.

- Do not automatically take herbs offered by traditional Chinese practitioners. They can interact with prescription drugs.

- Track your progress. If you have no response at all after four to six sessions, this therapy may not work for you. Or you may want to try another therapist because, as in any therapy, skill levels vary.[25]

Homeopathy

Homeopathy is a system of health care and treatment that was developed in the 1700s by Dr. Samuel Hahnemann. The philosophy of homeopathy is based on Dr. Hahnemann's research with natural medicines in which he found that "like cures like." A substance causing certain symptoms in a healthy person can cure a sick person with the same symptoms. This theory is based on the belief that the body enlists its own energies to heal itself and defend against illness. If a substance that causes symptoms similar to those of the illness is administered, the body steps up its fight against it, thereby promoting cure. This is known as the *law of similars*.

The substances may be made from plants such as aconite or dandelion; from minerals such as iron phosphate, arsenic oxide, or sodium chloride; from animals such as venom of a number of poisonous snakes, or the ink of the cuttlefish; or even from chemical drugs such as penicillin or streptomycin. These substances are diluted carefully until little of the original remains.

The National Center for Homeopathy (NCH) tells us that although most homeopathic medicines are available without a prescription, they are drug products made by homeopathic pharmacies, and their manufacture and sale are closely regulated by the federal Food and Drug Administration (FDA). Each individual state regulates the practice of homeopathy. Usually it can be employed legally by those whose degrees entitle them to practice medicine in that state. This includes the M.D. (medical doctor), D.O. (doctor of osteopathy), N.D. (doctor of naturopathy), D.D.S. (dentist), D.C. (doctor of chiropractic), and D.V.M. (veterinarian). Homeopathic practitioners can also include nurse practitioners, physician assistants, acupuncturists, and certified nurse midwives.[26]

Dr. Clifford Kearns, D.C., D.N.B.H.E., is a credentialed diplomat of the National Board of Homeopathic Examiners who practices homeopathy at Lutheran General Hospital's Center for Complementary Medicine in Park Ridge,

Resource Referral

To find a licensed practitioner near you, search the *National Center for Homeopathy* (NCH) *Membership Directory and Homeopathic Resource Guide,* or visit its Web site at www.homeopathic.org.

Illinois. Dr. Kearns believes that infertile couples can benefit greatly from the use of homeopathic remedies, but he cautions that successful results require the supervised guidance of a trained practitioner.

"Infertility is not solely a problem of the reproductive system," he says. "Homeopathy works through an understanding of the whole person. It is truly holistic medicine. The couple needs to learn why they have this problem and what is the root of the problem."

Dr. Kearns offers the example of a woman who adopted a 6-year-old girl after the girl's mother died. About 30 days after the death, the child started to show symptoms of hyperglycemia. Because the adoptive mom was a diabetic herself, she was familiar with the symptoms, brought her to be tested, and found that the child did have very high blood sugar levels. Dr. Kearns knows that a traditional medical doctor would begin to treat the little girl for juvenile diabetes (a chronic and debilitating condition) without considering the role that the intense psychic emotional insult the child had suffered might be playing in the development of the disease. In addition, the child had "patches" on her tongue and had become silent and reserved. All these factors combined dictated the homeopathic remedy that Dr. Kearns prescribed. After one dose of the remedy, the blood sugar returned to normal. One year later on the anniversary of the mother's death, the levels again rose; another dose brought them back down. Now at age 17, the girl has never had a recurrence of the diabetic symptoms. Dr. Kearns tells this story to explain why he believes the whole person, not just the symptoms, must be treated by a trained practitioner who will take several hours at the initial consultation to find out what is really going on.

> *Cliff Kearns, M.D., believes the whole person, not just the symptoms, must be treated by a trained practitioner who will take several hours at the initial consultation to find out what is really going on.*

"There are a million and one reasons why people struggle with infertility," says Dr. Kearns. "It can be endometriosis, low sperm count, or polycystic ovaries. Or, the problem can be rooted in financial stress, personal fears, and relationship troubles. There is no end to the possibilities. But the mind–body connection is definitely at work here. We're talking about a multifaceted problem with both physical and emotional dimensions. Infertility itself causes its own form of stress that further aggravates the problem.

"This all needs to be looked at from a global perspective," Dr. Kearns continues. "Who are you? What is your circumstance? What needs to be treated? For example, the homeopath in the initial 2-hour interview may discover that as an infertile woman, you are habitually tired, that you have 2 weeks of PMS each month, and you are overwrought and short-tempered with people you love. Through continued questioning, the practitioner may learn that you have cracks in the skin on the feet. This signals a homeopath that there is a hormone imbalance that can best be treated with the homeopathic remedy called sepia." You can see that because so many personal and medical factors are involved in proper homeopathic treatment, self-diagnosis and prescription make for a difficult and perhaps dangerous route.

A quick search by Dr. Kearns of a homeopathic database under the search term "sterility/infertility" brought up 204 possible remedies—each dependent on the total characteristics of the individual person. "One remedy will be for a woman who has a tendency not to retain semen in the reproductive tract (often loose-jointed people)," he says. "Others are for women with medical problems like endometriosis or polycystic ovaries. Still others are for men with sperm quality problems. There are also 166 remedies listed for women who conceive and then miscarry. Remedies in this category include those for women with anemia, fever, or anger; women with poor muscle tone in the genitals; women with coldness of the body, or constipation, or strong emotions. The list goes on and on, covering very specific and personal possible reasons for repeat miscarriages that can be treated with homeopathic remedies. These are all part of the whole picture that needs to be explored and cannot be uncovered in the 4.8 minutes allotted patients in traditional medical practices."

Herbs

Herbal remedies are no longer considered backstreet medicine in the United States. They are a rapidly growing, mainstream business— U.S. users spent an estimated $3.65 billion for herbal remedies in 1998, which was a 100 percent increase since 1994.[27] It is likely that you or your friends may have a few bottles of herbal supplements in your cabinet right now; advertisers tell us to buy *Ginkgo biloba* for brain power, St. John's wort for depression, and echinacea for colds and flu. And yes, some are recommended for the treatment of infertility symptoms. In fact, Dr. Ni reports that "different studies from China have suggested effectiveness in the areas of luteal phase defect, endometriosis, immunological infertility and male subfertility."[28]

Naturopathic physician Robin Dipasquale, N.D., is chair of the Botanical Medicine Department at Bastyr University in Washington and is in private practice in Duvall, Washington. Dr. Dipasquale uses a holistic approach to treating infertility that often includes the use of herbal remedies based on the couple's very individual needs. Although there are no herbs that claim to cure infertility, Dr. Dipasquale believes that some can address underlying problems that tend to sabotage the healthy functioning of the reproductive system. She will work with individuals who present with infertility concerns by assessing and treating other organ systems that may be out of balance and causing signs of anxiety, stress, ovarian dysfunction, menstrual dysfunction, or liver dysfunction.

> *Herbal remedies are no longer considered backstreet medicine in the United States. They are a rapidly growing, mainstream business.*

Herbs for Anxiety

Dr. Dipasquale is working with one woman who just found out that she is pregnant. "When she first came to me," she remembers, "it was clear that she was suffering from extreme anxiety after 17 years of not being able to give her husband a child. This anxiety was one of the leading pieces of her treatment plan."

When treating anxiety, Dr. Dipasquale begins with nerine herbs—a category of herbs that specifically supports the nervous system. In tea form, the nervines that Dr. Dipasquale uses include oats, lemon balm, kava, and scullcap, combined with oat straw. She believes that these herbs can make people feel generally calmer.

Herbs for Stress

As mentioned earlier, the state of the adrenal glands plays a strong role in the health of the reproductive system. The adrenal glands secrete cortisol during times of stress—the fight-or-flight hormone that can cause physical changes such as rapid heart rate, muscle tension, and increased blood pressure. If the building blocks or precursors for the production of hormones is utilized to produce cortisol, adequate precursors aren't available to produce reproductive hormones; thus, hormonal imbalances can result. Dr. Dipasquale uses a saliva test to check a person's cortisol level over a 24-hour period, which can tell her much about the function of the adrenal gland. Based on the results, she may prescribe herbs to assist in rebuilding the adrenal glands.

> *The herbs that are used to support and strengthen the functioning of the adrenal glands are called* adaptogens.

The herbs that are used to support and strengthen the functioning of the adrenal glands are called *adaptogens*. Among this group, the four that are frequently used to support fertility are Siberian ginseng, schizandra, devil's club, and licorice. (Licorice is not considered a true adaptogen herb, but it does prolong the half-life of cortisol in the body, allowing the adrenal glands to rest by not having to produce as much.)

"The effects of stress and anxiety," says Dr. Dipasquale, "on one's fertility are profound, yet the nervous and adrenal function are not usually attended to by conventional practitioners. I think it is very important."

Herbs for Ovarian Dysfunction

Many herbs can be mixed in formula to treat ovarian dysfunction. Three that stand out as specific for ovarian function are vitex, peony, and false unicorn root:

Vitex (also called *chasteberry*). This herb has the effect of stimulating and normalizing pituitary gland functions. (The pituitary gland will stimulate ovarian function, which then helps regulate the production and secretion of estrogen and progesterone.) Vitex can assist the pituitary gland to rebalance, which then signals the ovaries to function more optimally. It often can take 3 to 6 months before effects are recognized.

Peony (*Bai shao*). Peony's main job is to normalize ovarian function. It is used in combination with other herbs that support the ovaries to promote fertility. Peony's use comes from the Chinese herbal tradition.

False unicorn root (*Chamaelirium luteum*). This is a Western herb that normalizes and regulates ovarian function. False unicorn root is a plant identified by United Plant Savers as "at risk," endangered in its natural habitat, and difficult to grow under cultivation. Within the herbal community, practitioners are being asked to use an alternative choice. Peony may be a good substitute.

Herbs for Menstrual Dysfunction

To regulate a menstrual cycle, Dr. Dipasquale might use pituitary and hypothalamic glandular extracts or a biphasic hormonal formula.

Pituitary and hypothalamic glandular extracts. These are not botanicals, per se, but they are food for these glands in the brain that control the release and regulation of the reproductive hormones that control the menstrual cycle. These extracts nourish the glands, enabling them to function more effectively.

Biphasic hormonal formula. If Dr. Dipasquale sees that a woman's period is not regular, she will use different herbs in a biphasic formula to get the cycle back on schedule. In the first half of the month, she uses an estrogenic formula (supporting the estrogen phase of the cycle), and in the second half she'll use a progesterone formula (supporting the progesterone phase of the cycle). This can be effective in regulating the menstrual period in 3 to 6 months.

Herbs for Liver Function

The liver is the main organ of detoxification in the body. In addition to the foods and substances we consume, the liver processes our own metabolic waste products. All hormones, for example, move through the liver for processing before they are eliminated from the body. To summarize again, when the liver is functioning optimally, the "used" hormones are effectively removed, and the pituitary and hypothalamus in the brain are signaled to produce more. But if the liver function is weak (or stagnant), the "used" hormones remain in circulation, signaling the brain to slow down the production of new ones. This will throw off the hormonal balance required to support the reproductive system.

In addition to the foods and substances we consume, the liver processes our own metabolic waste products.

Because of this connection between liver function and reproductive hormones, Dr. Dipasquale often uses herbs that strengthen liver function. "There are many herbs used to tonify and move the liver," says Dr. Dipasquale. "The most commonly known one is dandelion root. Dandelion increases bile flow, assists with detoxification, and is rich in vitamins and minerals, especially vitamins A, D, C, and some of the Bs, iron, magnesium, zinc, and manganese."

A General Toner for Women

A Chinese herbal formula called Fertile Garden is used by Dr. Dipasquale as a general tonifying formula for women with fertility concerns or problems. It nurtures the yin of the kidneys (which means that it enhances the vital female energy and the moisture aspect), nurtures the yin of the liver (which means it helps with movement and flow and decreases tightness and constriction), and regulates the chi. This formula is generally available only through a certified herbalist or TCM practitioner.

An Herbal Remedy for Males

Scott Roseff, M.D., is a reproductive endocrinologist in private practice in West Orange, New Jersey, who recommends daily supplements of Pycnogenol brand French maritime pine bark extract for male subfertility. Frustrated by the high number of his patients with poor sperm parameters, Dr. Roseff began to investigate possible alternative solutions to this seemingly incurable problem.

"I began to read articles and studies that connected poor-quality sperm to the presence of oxygen-free radicals in the body," remembers Dr. Roseff. "These radicals are known to negatively affect cells; they can cause cellular damage and destruction and even tumors. We all have some degree of these radicals in our bodies from air pollution, water pollution, and environmental toxins and feel their effects in varying ways. Because sperm are cells, it is logical that they, too, are affected by oxygen-free radicals.

"After learning about the positive effects of certain antioxidants like vitamin C and E on these oxygen-free radicals," Dr. Roseff continues, "I became aware of an herbal supplement called Pycnogenol [Horphag Research Ltd., Switzerland], one of the most potent antioxidants known that comes from the bark of pine trees in France. I decided to conduct a study looking at the effect of this herbal therapy on sperm quality."

Dr. Roseff gave 200 milligrams daily of Pycnogenol to 19 men with poor sperm. "After 90 days, we found that the percentage of structurally normal sperm increased by an average of 99," he says. "We also did a sperm function test to evaluate the sperm's ability to bind to the egg and fertilize it; we again found significant improvement. And most importantly, most of the partners of the men in the study conceived."

Dr. Roseff's findings have been presented at numerous infertility conferences; the pilot study has already been published, and the final study is now under consideration for publication. Even though this is a small study that will undergo further investigation, the conclusions are noteworthy at a time when half of the infertility problems facing couples today are caused by poor-quality sperm—a problem handled in most conventional medical settings with the very expensive, time-consuming, and invasive in vitro fertilization. Dr. Roseff believes that by improving sperm quality, Pycnogenol can help many couples avoid IVF and enjoy natural conception or, at the very least, undergo less expensive and less invasive fertility-promoting procedures such as intra-uterine insemination.

Pycnogenol is available without a prescription in most stores that sell herbal products. Dr. Roseff recommends that for sperm treatment, the man take 1 milligram for each pound of body weight (so a 200-pound man would take 200 milligrams daily). Because men make new sperm only about every 3 months, it's important to take the supplement for at least that long before expecting results. Because there are no known negative side effects, and because antioxidants are good for general health improvement as well, this is a supplement men can continue to take without worry. But Dr. Roseff cautions that you should be careful to buy the product that lists Pycnogenol's patent number and pine tree symbol on the bottle to avoid the growing number of rip-off products that use their name but do not monitor quality. (Dr. Roseff can be reached via his Web site at www.reproendo.com.)

> *Scott Roseff, M.D., believes that by improving sperm quality, Pycnogenol can help many couples avoid IVF and enjoy natural conception or, at the very least, undergo less expensive and less invasive fertility-promoting procedures.*

Use Herbs with Caution

Despite the widespread belief, often fostered by advertising copy, that herbal preparations are "natural" and "drug-free," those that have druglike effects in the body do in fact contain potent chemicals that act like drugs, and they might have detrimental effects on men as well as women and might interfere with conception or a healthy pregnancy. This possibility prompted researchers at the Loma Linda University School of Medicine in Loma Linda, California, to explore the effects of four popular herbs on eggs and sperm.

Three of the herbs, St. John's wort, echinacea, and ginkgo, had ill effects on either eggs or sperm or both. The damage, the researchers said, included a reduced ability of sperm to penetrate an egg, changes to the genetic material in sperm, poor sperm viability, and, in the case of St. John's wort, mutation of the tumor suppressor gene, BRCA1, a change that can increase the risk of breast and ovarian cancers in women who inherit the mutated gene. Of the herbs tested, only saw palmetto, which is commonly taken by men to relieve the symptoms of an enlarged prostate, did not damage eggs or sperm in the doses tested. But even saw palmetto reduced the viability of sperm that were exposed to the herbal preparation for 7 days.

> *Herbs that have drug-like effects in the body do in fact contain potent chemicals that act like drugs, and they might interfere with conception or a healthy pregnancy.*

The researchers emphasized that their study, which was conducted in the laboratory on both human sperm and hamster eggs, indicated only a potential risk to those who take the herbs in question. They said it was possible that no untoward effects would occur in people who used the herbs in the usual recommended doses. However, the results do point to the potential negative effects herbs can have on infertility.[29]

This study gives you an idea of why herbs must be used with caution. Buying herbs off the shelf is risky business. Remember that the reproductive system of each person is unique from every other person. The choice of herbs that will be most helpful to you is based on your personal needs, general health status, and medical diagnosis. That's why choosing, formulating, and using herbs are best done under the guidance of a trained herbalist, TMC practitioner, or naturopathic physician who can individualize your herbal plan and also make sure that any herbs you take are absolutely safe for a woman even if she should become pregnant while taking them.

Unregulated Herbal Remedies

Be very careful when buying herbs off the shelf. Herbal remedy companies produce products that have never had any clinical testing and, because they are considered "food supplements" by the FDA, there are no controls regarding their purity, consistency, or effectiveness. There is no guarantee that what the label says is really in the bottle. Literature written by these companies is not subject to the stringent regulations that apply to pharmaceutical products.

Physical Therapy for Infertile Couples with Lower Back Pain

Nataly Pluta, P.T., Y.T., is a physical therapist and yoga therapist who has personally experienced the frustration of infertility and has found new hope in a common physical therapy technique called *myofascial release*. Pluta's interest in using physical therapy grew from her own difficulties as she navigated through the world of assisted reproductive technology. After surgical removal of a uterine fibroid that she was told was causing her infertility, Pluta still could not conceive. Then after finding that her husband had a low sperm count, she unsuccessfully underwent intrauterine inseminations with fertility medications, and on other occasions, tried donor sperm inseminations. Nothing worked and soon her fibroid returned. This one was also removed surgically, but it soon began to grow again. This frustrating process pushed Pluta to research a more natural approach to infertility.

"I knew that I had fibroids and that my husband had low sperm count," says Pluta, "but nobody could explain 'why.' So I began to more closely study anatomy and noticed that the nerves that innervate the lower back area were also those that fed into the reproductive system. Maybe it was no coincidence that my husband and I both had lower back pain and both had fertility problems. It was my belief that the impingement in the lumbar area was not only causing lower back pain; it obviously was blocking the nourishment from both the circulatory and nervous systems to the reproductive organs."

If you are infertile and also have lower back pain, Pluta suggests that you find a physical therapist who is trained in myofascial release and is open to the idea that freeing fascia in the pelvic area will improve nourishment to the reproductive system. This opinion does make sense: When a person has chronic pain, the connective tissue called the *fascia* is often involved. This tissue overlies each muscle and muscle fiber in the body. (You may have seen fascia if you take the skin off chicken before you cook it; it's that thin, clear layer of tissue between the skin and the meat.) Fascia is supposed to glide with us as we move, but emotional upset, physical trauma, or misalignment can cause the fascia to become dehydrated and inflexible. The fascia will then begin to bind together and impinge on the arteries and nerves, causing pain and restricted movement. The myofascial release technique for back pain and infertility is hands-on, deep-tissue work in the pelvic area to free up the flow of blood and nerve impulses to either the male or the female reproductive organs.

> *The myofascial release technique for back pain and infertility is hands-on, deep-tissue work in the pelvic area to free up the flow of blood and nerve impulses to either the male or the female reproductive organs.*

Sadly, Pluta and her husband have divorced since she began her research, but her fibroids have not returned, and she believes her reproductive health is much improved. She now runs workshops for infertile couples that combine myofascial release with yoga poses and chiropractic adjustments that promote pelvic circulation. (The stress-relieving benefit of yoga is discussed in chapter 6.) In these classes she has a 75 percent success rate of conception and full-term birth. "I'm not saying this is controlled scientific research or statistically significant," admits Pluta, "but those are the numbers I see, and many couples now have healthy children to show for it."

Manual Physical Therapy: The Wurn Technique

"About half of all female infertility cases may be helped through a new manual physical therapy and massage technique," says Larry Wurn, L.M.T., who, along with his wife Belinda Wurn, P.T., has pioneered and patented the Wurn Technique.

"These women are infertile due to mechanical (rather than medical or hormonal) causes," Wurn explains. "Mechanical infertility can be due to adhesions, which form as a result of the body's natural healing mechanism. As the body responds to inflammation, surgery, trauma, or infection, these adhesions can form on or near the delicate female reproductive organs and cause infertility. They may bind like a glue to the fingerlike fimbriae, preventing them from grasping the egg during ovulation. Adhesions may cling to the uterine surface, making it less receptive to the implantation of a fertilized egg. They can totally block the fallopian tubes, and they may also obstruct the healthy functioning of the ovaries."

These problems can be treated through medical surgeries, but Wurn believes that the Wurn Technique is a safer, less invasive alternative. According to Belinda Wurn, "No matter how skilled the physician, all surgeries, even laparoscopies, create adhesions. That's actually how the body heals from surgery. Surgical correction may also be temporary. For example, IVF and artificial inseminations are good only for one cycle. And most gynecologists agree that when fallopian tubes are opened surgically, they often close back up after a few weeks."

The Wurns have apparently been able to obtain more permanent results with their nonsurgical procedure; some of their patients have reported successive births in subsequent years, with no further therapy.

Working both externally and internally, they palpate the pelvic region, noting areas that feel thickened, warmer, less mobile, or "stuck." Then they use their hands to apply a very specific, gentle stretch to areas of abnormal tension in and around the body's muscles, organs, and connective tissues. Their focus is to restore normal structure, movement, and function by breaking down the adhesions, which tend to cover or glue down the delicate reproductive organs, impairing their ability to function normally. Women have attained full-term pregnancies after 5 to 23 hours of treatment.

The Wurns are now in the process of a clinical trial to give their work stronger scientific backing. Of the 20 women who have completed the trial so far, 14 have had full-term pregnancies or are presently pregnant. While this 70 percent success rate is very encouraging, the Wurns recognize that this study does not yet constitute rigorous scientific testing. It will be years until the results can be quantified in a multi-center study. However, as an alternative approach that is in no way harmful, the procedure offers much hope for women whose medical history indicates possible adhesion or microadhesion formation or poor biomechanics, and women whose infertility is unexplained. On their Web site, the Wurns state that any of the following may create an infertile condition that may be corrected through the Wurn Technique:

> *The Wurns's focus is to restore normal structure, movement, and function by breaking down the adhesions, which tend to cover or glue down the delicate reproductive organs, impairing their ability to function normally.*

- A history of infection or disease such as vaginal, bladder, kidney, liver, or yeast infections; endometriosis; appendicitis; pelvic inflammatory disease (PID); or sexually transmitted disease (STDs)

- A history of surgery such as a laparoscopy, appendectomy, D&C (dilation and curettage), abortion, surgical adhesion removal, "tummy tuck," cesarean, or episiotomy

- A history of trauma such as a slip and fall injury; falls onto the buttocks, hips, or back, or pelvic injury; or physical or sexual abuse

The Wurns know that using physical therapy to treat adhesions and increase reproductive function is a relatively new concept. "Your physician may have no direct knowledge or experience with this work," cautions Belinda. "It has only recently emerged as a therapeutic option, so most doctors are appropriately skeptical—and none are trained to perform the technique." At this time, the Wurns are the only practitioners in the country doing this technique, but they have received over a thousand letters from other therapists anxious to learn. The couple is now in the process of training other therapists from around the country and hope to license and certify 50 clinics within the next few years. In the meantime, you can contact them through their Web site at www.clearpassage.com or at their toll-free number, (866) BABYHERE.

> *The couple is now in the process of training other therapists from around the country and hope to license and certify 50 clinics within the next few years.*

PUTTING THE PIECES TOGETHER

Whether you want to use completely natural therapies to improve your state of fertility or want to use complementary and alternative therapies to improve your chances of a successful intrauterine insemination or in vitro fertilization, there are many possible options—even more than the ones discussed in this chapter. But which ones are best for you? Maybe you just need to better understand your own menstrual cycle and fertile times. Or, maybe your problem is caused by environmental toxins. Or, perhaps you need acupuncture to increase the flow of blood to your reproductive system. Or, maybe homeopathy or herbs would be best for you. Putting the pieces together can be an overwhelming challenge that leaves you trying a little of this and a little of that with little success. That's why, if you'd like to investigate these complementary and alternative approaches to infertility, you should contact a naturopathic physician. This is the person who can map out a personalized plan that is just right for you.

Like other naturopaths, Dr. Wynsome (who is a graduate of the Bastyr University Medical School in Seattle) uses an approach to treat

Look for the Real Thing

Naturopathic physicians are doctors. They attend medical school for 4 years like all other physicians. The first 2 years are spent alongside all other doctors-in-training, and then they all take the national board exam. Then, rather than going to a hospital to do rotations for the next 2 years, the naturopaths are trained in university clinics where they focus on natural therapeutics. However, the InterNational Council on Infertility Information Dissemination (INCIID) cautions, "Be fully aware of the credentials of any experts to whom you refer. A so-called 'certified naturopath' [naturpath or nutripath] can get his or her credentials for about $8,000 in home correspondence courses, and never have any clinical training."[30] Make sure the naturopath you choose is a licensed naturopathic primary care physician who has trained at an accredited naturopathic medical school.

infertility that is different than the one used by reproductive endocrinologists. "The reproductive endocrinologist is looking specifically at the egg and sperm and focusing on ovarian, tubal, or hormonal dysfunction," she says. "We are looking at a possible breakdown in multiple systems. We will work with the production and processing of hormones, nutrient deficiencies, toxic overload, metabolic function, and the health of the adrenal gland and the thyroid. We treat both men and women using safe, effective therapeutics—things like clinical nutrients, natural hormones, and herbal preparations that can all be used to support fertility. We can also integrate conventional medicine into the overall plan and thus are able to assist the patient in multiple approaches."

Some couples begin their search for answers with a naturopath because they do not want to get involved with invasive medical technology.

Others come to the naturopath as a last resort. "Often we see couples after they have unsuccessfully tried reproductive technologies," says Dr. Wynsome. "They've had IVF, GIFT, ZIFT, fertility medications, hormonal regulation, and so on, hoping for a 'quick' solution. Then they come to us and work on building optimal health for 2 to 4 months. Thirty to 35 percent of our patients will go on to conceive naturally; these numbers are just as good as those achieved by reproductive endocrinologists at the university hospitals. There are also others who will use naturopathic medicine to improve their level of fertility and then go on to successfully conceive through assisted reproductive technology." Either way, naturopathic physicians have a strong role to play in supporting a couple's desire to have a child.

TOTAL BODY HEALTH

Anne and her partner decided to have a baby when she was 36 years old. "I came from an extremely athletic background," she says, "and my monthly periods were not quite right, so before I even tried to conceive, I went directly to Dr. Wynsome to find out where I stood right from the start. I wanted to be in optimal health before I tried to carry a child through pregnancy."

Resource Referral

To find a naturopathic physician, contact the American Association of Naturopathic Physicians at (877) 969-2267 (or visit its Web site at www.naturopathic.org). Look specifically for doctors who specialize in infertility or endocrinology. You can also contact Dr. Wynsome at her clinic for a referral, an appointment, or further information at (206) 283-1383 or through her Web site at www.naturopathic.com.

Dr. Wynsome began by testing Anne's various hormonal levels and found that she was suffering adrenal exhaustion, evidenced by extremely high testosterone levels. "Dr. Wynsome had no doubt," remembers Anne, "that in this shape there was no way I was going to conceive a child. My progesterone and estrogen were not peaking at the time when I should have been ovulating, so I began to take low-dose natural progesterone to rebalance the hormones. Dr. Wynsome monitored the levels every 10 days or so and adjusted the dosage levels when necessary. I also gave myself a body tune-up to prepare for conception. With Dr. Wynsome's help, I went through a total fast detox. I uncovered all my food allergies and all my system weaknesses (I learned the liver was a little tired, and the kidneys needed support). I went on a very healthy, clean diet, and I made sure that I exercised every day."

At first the results were disappointing. Month after month there was still no pregnancy. At that point, Anne realized it was time to rethink her lifestyle to see whether her daily activities might be interfering with her level of fertility. "I'm a massage therapist," she says. "I was doing about 30 massages a week and commuting 10 miles each way every day by bicycle; at the same time, I was training 2 hours a day to be a yoga instructor and also training athletically for the cycling and kayaking that I love. I was going in high gear from 8 in the morning until 10 at night."

Anne suspected that her body might not be able to be this physically active and support a pregnancy, so something had to give.

Anne suspected that her body might not be able to be this physically active and support a pregnancy, so something had to give.

Anne recognizes that she may not be the typical infertility case due to her extremely high level of athleticism that may have caused the problem, but she does think there's an awful lot of women who are suffering the same effects of daily physical stress. "Women who are infertile and in their mid-30s or so are probably in midcareer," she says. "They most likely have dropped their cardiovascular workouts.

They face a lot of tension every day without the time or knowledge to deal with it. They rarely sleep or eat properly. Their bodies are just not able to recover, and this sets them up for fertility problems." Anne believes that all these lifestyle issues have to be addressed in order to have a healthy pregnancy.

"For the next 6 months," says Anne, "I got really serious about making this work. I stopped taking the progesterone for a while and cut down on all the high-end stressors in my day. I cut my work hours, and I stopped my daily workout and weight lifting completely. My body needed a rest." At this same time, Anne visited an acupuncturist at Dr. Wynsome's suggestion. After only three sessions, Anne's menstrual cycle returned to a normal pattern.

"When I felt my body was ready, I went back on the progesterone and really put a lot of attention on my menstrual cycle," Anne says. "I kept close watch on my basal body temperature. Because my uterus tips backward, we changed our sex position, and after sex I did a yoga shoulder stand to let gravity facilitate the process. With the odds already against me, I figured any small thing I could do to raise the odds was worth it."

It certainly was worth it when, at age 41, Anne became pregnant and nine months later delivered a healthy 9-pound, 8-ounce baby boy. His dad, Harry, says, "Our baby has inherited his mom's smile and sweet temperament, and my name and (hopefully) good taste in women."

Looking back, Anne is very glad she chose a natural route. "For me, my naturopathic physician played the role of a coach," she says. "She told me, 'Here are the facts. This is what's going on in your body and here's why. These are the options you have. If you choose this option, this is the best way to make it work.' I felt very involved in what was happening to me. I was active in bringing my own body into a state where conception and a healthy pregnancy could occur naturally. I felt that genetically, as a female, it was my job to reproduce, but like many infertile women, I had done something to freak my body out so it just didn't want to do it. Technically, I shouldn't have become pregnant and delivered this wonderful baby, but I did, and I think that happened because I took the time to get my body in good shape with the guidance of a wonderful naturopathic physician."

MOVING ON

The natural approach to fertility has successfully given children to thousands of couples who were told they were infertile. Many of these therapies are proven safe and highly effective. But they are not successful for everyone. Many infertile couples need more conventional, and sometimes invasive, medical treatments to help them conceive and deliver a child. These treatments are explained in the next chapter.

CHAPTER 4

Medical Infertility Treatments

IF YOU'VE HIT many a dead-end in your travels through the infertility maze, there's good news on the treatment front: According to the American Society for Reproductive Medicine (ASRM), recent improvements in medication, microsurgery, and in vitro fertilization (IVF) techniques make pregnancy possible for more than half of the couples pursuing treatment.[1] The last 5 years alone have brought big changes in treating infertility and in assisting couples who want to conceive.

This chapter will give you an overview of the treatment options available today, divided into two main categories: restoring or bringing about fertility and assisted reproductive technology (ART). Seeing all the possibilities listed in black and white will help you better understand the decisions you may have to make, how to proceed, and what to expect once you get going. Having this information lets you become a more active participant in the creation of your future family. So stay involved, ask questions, and choose what's best for you.

RESTORING OR BRINGING ABOUT FERTILITY

Often there are identifiable reasons for infertility. The female may have an abnormal menstrual cycle that needs to be regulated; the male may have an obstruction that blocks the passage of sperm. These types of problems can often be rectified and fertility restored. In fact, the ASRM says that 85 to 90 percent of infertility cases are treated with conventional medical therapies such as medication or surgery.[2] This section will take a look at treatment options for some of the most common medical causes of infertility in both females and males.

Treatment Options for Common Medical Problems in Females

The treatment possibilities discussed here are most often suggested for younger women who have time to correct the abnormality and still conceive naturally. Women in their 40s, however, are often advised to skip these treatment options and move their treatment plan directly to some method of ART. If you are in your late 30s or in your 40s, it's understandable that you may not want to take the time to undergo treatment, wait for your body to heal or regulate, and then try natural conception (which even for the general fertile population under 30 years old offers only a 20 percent chance of conception each month). Your choice, of course, depends on your medical condition, your age, and your doctor's recommendation. The following information will give you the facts you need to make an educated decision.

Treatment for Ovulatory Disorders

The failure to ovulate (release eggs) will prevent the normal process of conception. If you have missing or irregular menstrual periods, you are likely to have some kind of ovulatory disorder, which can be caused by a number of conditions. If you have ovulatory problems due to a hormonal imbalance, fertility medications (as explained later in this chapter) can restore the balance.

One particular ovulatory disorder that can cause infertility is called *polycystic ovary syndrome* (PCOS). PCOS is characterized by many enlarged, smooth ovarian cysts, as well as an abnormal menstrual cycle. To reverse infertility in women with PCOS, doctors frequently start with fertility drug treatment (described in the next section) to regulate ovulation. If, however, the ovaries have large cysts on them, some fertility specialists may want to cauterize the ovary through laparoscopic surgery. Roughly 62 percent of PCOS women who undergo this procedure successfully go on to conceive; when the surgery is combined with fertility drug therapy, the pregnancy rates are as high as 80 percent.[3] That is good news!

Some women with polycystic ovaries have irregular ovulation due to glucose intolerance (more specifically, insulin resistance). They can be tested by doing a fasting blood sugar and a fasting insulin level and also a full glucose tolerance test. If there is an abnormality, such as a subclinical diabetic condition or just abnormal lab results, the women may benefit from treatment with oral hypoglycemics. The drugs in this class (such as metformin) can be used to regulate the menstrual cycles and lead to ovulatory cycles without using any fertility drugs. Even if these drugs fail to cause regular menstrual cycles, they can be combined with oral fertility drugs (such as clomiphene citrate) to effect results where oral fertility drugs alone would not work well.

Fertility Drug Treatment

Fertility drugs are the primary treatment for women who are infertile due to ovulation disorders. To better understand why these drugs are an almost-standard part of infertility treatment, let's review how the different hormones in the body naturally affect the reproductive cycle.

The follicle-stimulating hormone (FSH) is primarily responsible for stimulating growth of the ovarian follicle, which includes the developing egg, the cells surrounding the egg that produce the hormones needed to support a pregnancy, and the fluid around the egg. As the follicle grows, an increasing amount of the hormone estrogen is produced by the cells in the follicle and released into the bloodstream. Estrogen causes the endometrium (lining of the uterus) to thicken before ovulation occurs. The higher blood levels of estrogen will also tell the hypothalamus and pituitary gland in the brain to slow the production and release of FSH.

The luteinizing hormone (LH) also helps increase the amount of estrogen produced by the follicle cells. However, its main function is to cause ovulation. The sharp rise in the blood level of LH that triggers ovulation is called the *LH surge*. After ovulation, the group of hormone-producing follicle cells become the corpus luteum, which will produce estrogen and large amounts of another hormone, progesterone. Progesterone causes the endometrium to mature so that it can support implantation of the fertilized egg or embryo. If implantation of a fertilized egg does not occur, the levels of estrogen and progesterone decrease, the endometrium sloughs off, and menstruation occurs.[4]

When this reproductive sequence does not happen properly, fertility drugs can help. They may be used as the sole method of treatment, or they may be used to support an ART procedure such as in vitro fertilization. The most commonly used fertility drugs are the following:

Clomiphene citrate (Clomid, Serophene, Milophene). This drug is used to stimulate ovulation. It causes the pituitary gland to release more FSH and LH, which stimulates the growth of an egg follicle.

Human menopausal gonadotropin, hMG (Pergonal, Humegon, Repronex). This medication is prescribed for women who don't menstruate on their own due to the failure of the pituitary gland to stimulate ovulation. Unlike clomiphene, which stimulates the pituitary gland, hMG and other gonadotropins directly stimulate the ovaries.

Human chorionic gonadotropin, or hCG (Perganyl). Used in combination with clomiphene citrate, hMG, and FSH, this drug stimulates the follicle to release its egg.

FSH (Follistim, Gonal-F). FSH is essentially hMG without LH. Like hMG, it works by stimulating the ovaries to mature egg follicles.

Gonadotropin-releasing hormone, or GnRH (Factrel, Lutrepulse). This medication is used in women whose hypothalamus doesn't properly release the natural hormone GnRH, which stimulates the pituitary gland's release of FSH and LH. GnRH is administered in a pattern that mimics the natural rhythm by use of a pump that is connected to your vein or fat tissue.

GnRH analogs (Lupron, Synarel, Zoladex). These drugs are used in conjunction with fertility drugs to prevent premature ovulation (before the lead follicle is mature enough) during hMG treatment.

Bromocriptine (Parlodel). This medication is used to treat women whose ovulation cycles are irregular due to elevated levels of prolactin, the hormone that stimulates milk production in new mothers. Bromocriptine inhibits prolactin production.[5]

Progesterone. Progesterone is prescribed to prepare the uterus to support the implantation of the fertilized eggs (embryos).

Risks of Fertility Drugs

The medications used to promote fertility are usually very well tolerated. However, as with all medical treatments, there are some potential problems you should be aware of.

Ovarian hyperstimulation syndrome. This condition can occur whenever women use any fertility drug or ovarian stimulation medications, especially injectable gonadotropins. When severe, ovarian

---

No More Injections?

The drug Crinone is available in gel form and can be used in place of injectable progesterone. It is administered vaginally once or twice daily using a prefilled, disposable applicator. In a recent study of 2,000 women in 23 infertility treatment centers throughout the United States, the gel was equally effective as the injected form in helping women achieve pregnancy.[6] Other vaginal applications of progesterone such as progesterone vaginal capsules or suppositories can be as effective when used twice daily.

hyperstimulation can lead to dehydration, large amounts of fluid accumulation in the abdominal and lung cavities, blood clotting disorders, and kidney damage. Rarely, IVF cycles are canceled to prevent hyperstimulation. (In this case, the embryos are frozen rather than transferred.) Severe hyperstimulation requiring hospitalization occurs in less than 1 percent of women who have egg retrieval with IVF.[7]

Fertility drugs and multiple births. Fertility drugs are responsible for multiple births in 20 to 40 percent of all conceptions due to their use. (Twins represent the overwhelming majority of multiple pregnancies.) While clomiphene citrate only rarely results in pregnancy with more than twins, hMG and FSH carry a greater risk of causing higher-order multiples. About 25 percent of hMG and FSH treatment cycles result in multiple pregnancies—about two-thirds being twins and one-third being triplets or more.[8] However, using hMG and FSH in IVF cycles only actually controls higher-order multiples and reduces their incidence to less than 10 percent by restricting the number of embryos transferred.

Multiple births add a degree of risk to the pregnancy: As a rule, the greater the number of fetuses, the higher the risk of premature labor. (Babies born prematurely are at increased risk of a number of medical and developmental problems.) Multiples also increase the risk of maternal hemorrhage, cesarean delivery, pregnancy-induced high blood pressure, gestational diabetes, and lower birth weight.

In some cases, the risk of multiple pregnancies can be reduced. If a woman requires an hCG injection to trigger ovulation and ultrasound exams show that too many follicles have developed, she and her physician can decide to withhold the hCG injection. Or, if too many babies are conceived, the removal of one or more fetuses (multiple pregnancy reduction) can offer improved survival odds for the surviving fetuses. However, this presents serious emotional and ethical challenges for many people. Couples considering fertility drug treatment should discuss this possibility with their doctors before starting therapy. (You'll find more details on the debate over multiples in chapter 7.)

Possible cancer risk. Some studies have suggested a link between clomiphene citrate and an increased, long-term risk of developing ovarian tumors if more than 12 cycles of treatment were done. Injectable medications (hMG, FSH) have not been associated with this problem. In 1998, a large study followed more than 10,000 women who had undergone in vitro fertilization between 1978 and 1992. Slightly more than half had been treated with at least one cycle of fertility drugs; the other women had not. The study found no difference in the incidence of ovarian cancer between the two groups during the time period. Research is ongoing on this issue. This also may be an important topic to discuss with your doctor before initiating treatment with fertility drugs.[9]

Ectopic pregnancy. *Ectopic* (tubal) *pregnancies* are those in which the fertilized egg implants itself outside the uterus, usually in the fallopian tubes. This occurs in 1 to 2 percent of pregnancies in the general population; the rate is slightly increased for those women taking ovulatory stimulating drugs. The ectopic pregnancy rate is anywhere from 25 to 35 percent in the general infertile population conceiving by non-IVF methods. IVF is a safer alternative in these cases.

Treatment for Uterine Problems

Some cases of infertility are caused by abnormalities in the woman's uterus. The diagnostic hysterosalpingogram, sonohysterogram (hysterosonogram), and hysteroscopy can find many of these problems and often they can be corrected through surgery if needed. If you remember Penny in chapter 1, she had surgery to remove a septum in her uterus, which is a thin wall of tissue that doctors felt was causing her repeat miscarriages. Other uterine problems, such as polyps, fibroids, and scarring of the uterine cavity, can be corrected without even making an abdominal surgical incision. Under anesthesia, a small instrument (a hysteroscope) that is connected to a light source is inserted through the cervix and into the uterus. Small surgical instruments such as scissors, lasers, and a variety of other instruments can then be introduced to correct the abnormalities. Surgical corrections of uterine abnormalities may dramatically increase the chances of a successful pregnancy.

Treatment for Tubal Disorders

Damaged fallopian tubes can cause infertility. These organs may be damaged due to a birth defect; a number of traumas such as a burst appendix, abdominal surgery, or infection after abortion; or surgery to remove a tubal pregnancy. More commonly, fallopian tubes are damaged by a previous infection, such as a sexually transmitted disease (often gonorrhea or chlamydia) or pelvic inflammatory disease (PID).

Microsurgical techniques often permit blockages or other problems in the fallopian tubes to be repaired. Surgical repair offers a 10 to 30 percent chance of achieving a successful pregnancy.[10] But keep in mind that although surgical repair can technically open tubes, tissue damage due to prior insults cannot be healed or corrected. Also, because the pregnancy rate after surgery is rather low, and an extended period of time must be allowed for healing and the restoration of the

> *Surgical repair offers a 10 to 30 percent chance of achieving a successful pregnancy.*

menstrual cycle, age can become a deciding factor in choosing this surgery. Women who are in their late 30s or in their 40s will often opt to bypass a tubal problem by using some form of IVF (which also has a protective advantage due to the lower incidence of ectopic pregnancy).

Tubal Ligation Reversals

Some women are infertile because they had their fallopian tubes surgically "tied" to prevent pregnancy. Life circumstances such as divorce or death of a spouse and then remarriage sometimes send these women back to their surgeons in the hopes of reversing the sterility procedure. In the past, the surgery was a major event, and the reversal rates were low. Gary S. Berger, M.D., of the Chapel Hill Tubal Reversal Center in North Carolina, says that the kind of abdominal surgery still typically performed around the country causes tissue trauma, postoperative pain, and the need for narcotic medications, immobilization, and several days of post-op hospitalization, as well as a 6-week recovery period.

However, thanks to newer microsurgical techniques, the reversal can be accomplished without nerve blocks, pain, bleeding, immobilization, narcotic medications, and post-op hospitalization. Dr. Berger has specialized in this technique for the past 25 years and has performed over 2,000 such procedures on an outpatient basis. "My patients," says Dr. Berger, "typically are alert, dressed, and walking around within 90 minutes after surgery, and they can then be discharged to recover at home. This decreases the cost to the patient by one-half to three-fourths, as compared to performing the procedure on an in-patient basis. The average recovery time until returning to full activities is 7 to 10 days instead of the usual 6 weeks."

Although Dr. Berger recognizes that the success of tubal ligation reversal varies with the age of the woman (in fact, the procedure is not recommended for women over 38 because IVF gives quicker results), the methods that were used for the tubal sterilization, and the methods that are used for the reversal, he says, "For women of similar ages and methods of tubal sterilization, microsurgical techniques have been shown to be about twice as effective as nonmicrosurgical techniques—pregnancy rates of 70 to 90 percent compared with 35 to 45 percent for women who are ovulating normally and are not perimenopausal." For more information on the microsurgery technique of tubal ligation reversal, see Dr. Berger's Web site at www.tubalreversal.net.

> *Thanks to newer microsurgical techniques, the reversal can be accomplished without nerve blocks, pain, bleeding, immobilization, narcotic medications, and post-op hospitalization.*

Treatment for Endometriosis

In some women, wayward endometrial cells implant themselves outside the uterus on any structure, including the ovaries, fallopian tubes, bladder, bowel, and the lining of the abdominal cavity. This condition is called *endometriosis*, and it can cause a number of conditions related to infertility, including pelvic adhesions, distorted anatomy, and ovarian or tubal damage. In addition, the ovulatory process may be disturbed.[11]

Unfortunately, infertility due to endometriosis is often difficult to treat. Although hormone medications are effective for treating the disease itself, they are not very useful for treating the infertility caused by endometriosis because they temporarily turn off ovarian function—not very helpful if you want to become pregnant! Doctors have found some success by removing the implants through laparoscopic surgery. This is followed by superovulation therapy with fertility drugs and sometimes in vitro fertilization. It is encouraging that about 40 percent of women who have an operative laparoscopy procedure will go on to conceive.[12] Before you opt for this surgery, however, keep in mind that minimal endometriosis, if untreated, allows for the same pregnancy rates as cases treated.

> *About 40 percent of women who have an operative laparoscopy procedure will go on to conceive.*

Treatment for Recurrent Miscarriage

Blood tests may reveal the possible reason for repeat miscarriages and give the doctor a reasonable course of treatment. Because repeat miscarriages are known to be caused by hormonal imbalances, antiphospholipid antibodies, thyroid disease, and diabetes, you will be tested for all these conditions. If any of the blood tests are positive, appropriate medication will be prescribed to treat the condition and possibly restore fertility.

Sometimes surgery is necessary if any anatomical problems are detected in the reproductive tract. As explained earlier, many uterine abnormalities can be surgically corrected. For example, another anatomical problem known to cause premature delivery in the second trimester is an incompetent cervix. The cervix is supposed to stay tightly closed until time of birth, but in some cases it malfunctions and releases the baby too soon. An incompetent cervix can be diagnosed by history, x ray, and other simple procedures and can be surgically managed.

Treatment Options for Common Medical Problems in Males

The treatment options for male infertility focus on improving the number and quality of sperm. Your doctor will first diagnose the cause of sperm abnormalities (if possible) and then decide whether any of the following treatments are appropriate.

Medication

Medication is sometimes used to treat infertility caused by antisperm antibodies or infection. It can also (but not often successfully) be used to correct sperm deficiencies. When sperm production is impaired because of damage to the sperm-producing areas of the testicles, drug treatment has been of little use. But in extremely rare instances when sperm production is hampered because of a pituitary problem, treatment with hormone medications may help.[13] Human chorionic gonadotropin, for example, can elevate the amount of testosterone to the correct level. In addition, you may be given injectable gonadotropins or clomiphene citrate. These medications are used to help women develop eggs in their ovaries, but they are also used as fertility medicines to help men with low sperm counts produce more sperm.

Treatment for Retrograde Ejaculation

When the bladder neck doesn't close as it should when a male ejaculates, the seminal fluid is propelled backward into the bladder instead of continuing down the urethra and out the tip of the penis. When this happens, semen is then mixed with the urine in the bladder, where the acidity of the urine kills the sperm, which are then excreted during urination. This condition is called *retrograde ejaculation*.

Eric Seaman, M.D., attending surgeon in urology at St. Barnabas Medical Center in New Jersey, says the treatment for retrograde ejaculation includes the use of medication and then collection of sperm from the bladder. "The patient will first take medication before he has an ejaculation to alkalinize the urine [reduce the level of acidity]. We may also introduce into the bladder some kind of buffer solution that will keep the pH level constant. After he ejaculates, he will then urinate into a cup to pass the sperm, which is now hopefully still living because the urine is not highly acidic. This sperm can then be used in various ART procedures.

"Some men will also try medications that help tighten up the bladder neck muscles. Certain cold medications [i.e., sympathominetics] can be used for this purpose because they increase the body's sympathetic nervous system that can tighten up these muscles." Dr. Seaman says that if the sperm do not exit with the urine, there is still hope. The doctor can retrieve the sperm by passing a catheter up the urethra into the bladder.

Treatment for Varicoceles: Varicocelectomy

The majority of men with varicoceles (varicose veins in the scrotum) remain fertile and asymptomatic. Therefore, treatment of all varicoceles is clearly unnecessary. According to Jean Fourcroy, M.D., Ph.D., from the Uniformed Services University of Health Sciences in Bethesda, Maryland, "Repair of the varicocele is indicated when the couple has documented infertility, the female is normal or potentially fertile, the male has one or more abnormal semen parameters, and there is the presence of a varicocele on physical examination."

> *Varicocelectomy usually can be done on an outpatient basis and is relatively free of complications.*

Treatment, if needed to improve fertility or to decrease scrotal swelling, is primarily surgical. During a varicocelectomy, the dilated veins are tied off (ligated) through a small incision in the scrotum. This procedure usually can be done on an outpatient basis and is relatively free of complications. There is a slight risk of infection any time an incision is made, but this risk is minimal. The discomfort is not usually disabling and clears in a few days. Long-term adverse effects are exceedingly rare. Using the microsurgical technique employed at Cornell, Marc Goldstein, M.D., and Peter Schlegel, M.D., have reviewed the results of over 1,500 men who underwent microsurgical varicocelectomy. The couples' pregnancy rate was 43 percent after 1 year and 69 percent after 2 years, compared to 16 percent in couples with men who declined surgery and had hormonal treatment or used insemination.[14] Although this procedure has been helpful in improving sperm number and motility, it does not help if sperm morphology (shape) is abnormally low.

Treatment for Obstruction: Epididymostomy

If you have an anatomical obstruction that blocks the passage of sperm through the epididymis, the obstructed area can be bypassed through microsurgery. This is the same surgery that is used to reverse a vasectomy.

Alternately, sperm could be microsurgically aspirated with a very small-gauge needle under local anesthesia. The collected sperm can then be used for sperm injection during in vitro fertilization of harvested eggs.

Vasectomy Reversal

Vasectomy is one of the most common operations performed today in the United States (about one-quarter of a million men undergo this operation every year), and it is the most popular method of birth control in the world.[15] For as many reasons as men choose to have a vasectomy, others choose to have the vasectomy reversed. If infertility is the result of a vasectomy, thanks to advances in microsurgery, the chances of successful reversal are quite good.

During a vasectomy, the vas deferens (which is the tube that carries the sperm from the epididymis to the prostate gland) is severed during a 5-minute surgery in the doctor's office under local anesthesia. It is not difficult to identify and cut the vas deferens with its fairly thick (about $1/8$th of an inch) diameter and tough outer muscular wall. A vasectomy reversal, however, is much more difficult because of the microscopic

> *If infertility is the result of a vasectomy, thanks to advances in microsurgery, the chances of successful reversal are quite good.*

size of the inner canal within the vas deferens that carries the sperm. The diameter of this inner canal is about $1/70$th to $1/100$th of an inch, or roughly the size of a pinpoint. This inner canal has a lining, which is about three cells thick, approximately $1/2,000$th of an inch. Obviously, then, it is not so easy to reattach these tiny structures in working order.

In the not-to-distant past of the 1970s, vasectomy reversals were successful only about 25 percent of the time—even when the reconnection was completed successfully. It was then discovered that over time, a vasectomy causes a blockage due to pressure damage closer to the testicles, in the epididymis, that prevents sperm from ever reaching the vasectomy site. Today, extremely refined microsurgical techniques can either repair or bypass the damaged area. Now, the success rate of vasectomy reversals is close to 90 percent.[16]

Fertility does not return immediately after a vasectomy reversal. All of the old sperm that have been stored up over the years since the vasectomy have died of old age. This dead sperm material must be cleaned out after the vasectomy is reversed to make room for the new sperm, which usually do not appear for about 3 months or more. Usually if the microsurgery is performed well, most men are fertile within a year and their partner is pregnant within 2 years.

ASSISTED REPRODUCTIVE TECHNOLOGY (ART)

Some infertile couples cannot or do not have time to medically restore fertility and conceive a child naturally. But with a little assistance from modern technology, they can still become natural parents. In fact, to date over 70,000 American babies have been born thanks to advances in assisted reproductive technologies (ART).[17] The methods of ART discussed in this chapter include artificial insemination and in vitro fertilization (IVF).

ART cannot work miracles, however. It works best when the woman has a healthy uterus, responds well to fertility drugs, and ovulates naturally or uses donor eggs, and the man has healthy sperm or

Vocabulary 101

Before you go any further, here are some terms you need to know so you don't get totally lost in medical lingo:

Gamete: the male and female reproductive cells—the sperm (spermatozoon) and the egg (ovum)

Oocyte: the immature ovum, the unfertilized female gamete or sex cell (egg) produced in the ovaries each month, that contains the genetic information to be transmitted by the female

Zygote: an egg that has been fertilized but not yet divided

Blastocyst: a fertilized egg that has divided to 80 to 100 cells usually over 5 days

Embryo: the developing baby from implantation to the second month of pregnancy

In vitro: a term meaning "outside the human body; in an artificial environment"

In vivo: a term meaning "within the body"

donor sperm are available. When donor eggs or sperm are not used, there's a lower success rate in women older than 42, in women faced with early menopause who no longer produce as many eggs, and in women with untreated conditions of the uterus, such as scar tissue.

Artificial Insemination (AI)

Artificial insemination is a process in which sperm are collected and processed, and then placed inside the woman for the purpose of producing a pregnancy. This form of ART may work in cases of retrograde ejaculation (ejaculation into the bladder instead of the penis), premature or delayed ejaculation, poor sperm quality or low count, and unexplained infertility. Along with fertility drugs, it is often the first method of ART recommended to couples as long as the female partner has open tubes.

The most commonly used type of insemination is called *intrauterine insemination* (IUI). In this procedure, the sperm are placed into the woman's uterus. Other less common methods include *intracervical insemination* (ICI), in which the sperm are placed into the cervical canal, and *intratubal insemination* (ITI), in which the sperm are placed into the fallopian tubes.

The reason for the popularity of IUI over the other methods was highlighted by a research team composed of scientists at the National Institutes of Child Health and Human Development's National Cooperative Reproductive Medicine Network, headed by David S. Guzick, M.D., Ph.D., of the University of Rochester in New York. They conducted a study to give couples and doctors general statistical guidelines to evaluate a series of common insemination treatments.

> *The most commonly used type of insemination is called intrauterine insemination (IUI). In this procedure, the sperm are placed into the woman's uterus.*

In all, the investigators tested 932 couples with infertility in which the woman appeared to ovulate normally, including those having unexplained infertility and those with less severe forms of male factor infertility. The couples who took part in the study were assigned to one of four groups:

Group 1. In the control group, the women did not receive any drugs to induce ovulation and were inseminated in the cervix (ICI). Insemination took place when the woman's urinary levels of LH peaked.

Group 2. These women did not receive any drugs to induce ovulation but were inseminated in the uterus with sperm (IUI) when their urinary levels of LH peaked.

Group 3. These women received injections of FSH to induce them to ovulate and then received ICI.

Group 4. These women received FSH injections and IUI.

The 231 women in the fourth group receiving FSH injections and IUI had the highest rate of pregnancy at 33 percent. In comparison, the 234 couples receiving induced ovulation and ICI had a pregnancy rate of 19 percent. The 234 women receiving IUI timed to coincide with a surge in LH had a pregnancy rate of 18 percent, and the 233 women receiving ICI timed to surge in LH had a pregnancy rate of 10 percent. "Clearly," said coauthor Dr. Donna Vogel, "treatment with induced ovulation and intrauterine insemination is more effective in this population than any of the other methods we tested. This information is particularly important in view of the high costs of the procedures involved—induced ovulation, for example, averages about $1,300 per cycle."[18]

You and your doctor will decide which procedure is best for you based on your unique personal needs. The majority of women take a combination of fertility medications before insemination to prompt the ovaries to make multiple eggs, thus improving their chances of getting one (or more) to fertilize. However, sometimes the ovaries become overstimulated and far too many eggs are produced. In this case, it is too risky to proceed with the insemination and risk higher-order multiple embryos. The insemination will be canceled and attempted again a month or two later, usually with a reduced dose of medication.

> *The majority of women take a combination of fertility medications before insemination to prompt the ovaries to make multiple eggs, thus improving their chances of getting one (or more) to fertilize.*

If you should be in danger of having an insemination cycle canceled because of ovarian overstimulation, ask your doctor about a procedure called FASIAR (follicular reduction/intraperitoneal insemination) that allows the insemination cycle to continue even when the ovaries have been overstimulated. In this procedure, a needle aspiration is used to remove some of the eggs before the sperm are flushed in. "Basically," says Eric Scott Sills, M.D., a reproductive endocrinologist with the Georgia Reproductive Specialists in Atlanta, "we are reducing the number of eggs and then inserting sperm directly into the body to fertilize

Angela and Shawn: Still Holding onto Hope

When 34-year-old Angela and her 39-year-old husband Shawn, who have been married 8 years, were unable to conceive a second child, they decided to give artificial insemination a try. Since that decision 3 years ago, they have been riding the emotional ups and downs of infertility.

"I had no problem conceiving Kyle 7 years ago," remembers Angela. "I went off the pill and one month later was pregnant! That's why it's so hard to understand why I'm having so much trouble now." When Angela didn't become pregnant again after trying for 18 months, her obstetrician gave her a prescription for Clomid and told her to relax and have a bottle of wine and everything would be fine. Four months later, Angela still was not pregnant, and her hysterosalpingogram showed no abnormalities. This is when Angela made her first appointment with a reproductive endocrinologist.

This doctor prescribed more Clomid and suggested an artificial insemination. This sounded like a real positive step, but, unfortunately, the insemination was unsuccessful—as were the following four inseminations with Clomid. The doctor then suggested a diagnostic laparoscopy. Angela had the surgery and found nothing was wrong. Moving to the next level, Angela agreed to try another insemination but this time using injectable drugs. She began self-injecting a drug called Follistim to stimulate the ovaries to make mature egg follicles.

"My husband did not want me to do this at all," says Angela. "I begged him to agree to just 3 months (which we later stretched to 4), and he went along with it, but he hates needles and wasn't going to be able to help me administer them." Angela injected herself in the stomach each evening for five nights. A close friend who is a nurse agreed to give her the injection in her buttocks that was needed at the end to release the egg. Three times during that week, Angela went back to the doctor's office for monitoring by blood tests and ultrasound to make sure the ovaries were not being over stimulated. "I got all bruised from the shots," Angela remembers, "but it seemed worth it when they told me that my eggs were perfect, the numbers were good, and this time it was going to work."

When the egg was released, Shawn gave his sperm donation at home in a little container, and Angela took it to the doctor's office. "My husband stayed at home to take care of Kyle while I took 'the boys' in and then waited an hour and a half while they were processed. The insemination itself is really no big deal. It felt kind of like getting a Pap smear. They inserted the sperm up into the uterus, and then I just laid there for about 15 minutes before getting up. Then it was done, I went home, and the wait began."

Waiting is the hard part. "It's so tempting to get excited," says Angela. "But you learn not to get your hopes up. I'd rather expect the worst and be surprised if I'm wrong than be let down again."

Nobody has to tell a woman the insemination didn't work; the failure is announced when the menstrual bleeding begins. "Nobody I know who is struggling with infertility bothers with at-home pregnancy tests," says Angela. "We all know our bodies so well, we know exactly what's going on in our reproductive cycle minute by minute. I can tell you at any given time what day it is in my cycle. Women who are fertile have no idea; they don't have to monitor themselves so carefully."

Angela has been let down over and over again. In all, five times she used Clomid with insemination and three times she used injectable drugs with insemination, and all eight times the approach has failed. After the last failure, she went to another reproductive endocrinologist for a second opinion. He immediately diagnosed polycystic ovarian syndrome, a common cause of infertility that had been missed by her two previous doctors. Now Angela has new hope and

(continues)

(continued)

feels optimistic about her ability to be more actively involved in what will happen in the future.

"I know now that the more informed you are, the better," she says. "In the beginning I went into this blindly, figuring that the doctors know what's best for me. Now I know what diagnostic tests I should have had, and I know I should never have taken Clomid for so many months and wasted all that time and put myself through 12 months of up-and-down hell. Now I research and make up a list of questions that I bring to my doctor visits. I feel much better about myself and where we're going with this. I still have hope." (Angela and Shawn's hope has paid off. After receiving treatment for her PCOS, Angela conceived a child through the old-fashioned, natural method, and as this book goes to press, she is 24 weeks pregnant.)

the ones that remain. This reduces the cost, but it is definitely not widely performed.

"Nobody starts out planning to do a FASIAR procedure," Dr. Sills adds. "It is a creative way to avoid having to cancel an intrauterine insemination cycle and stop treatment because of a very high response to ovulation induction. It's like a medical reduction of follicles so there aren't 20 eggs waiting to be fertilized."

In Vitro Fertilization

In vitro fertilization (IVF) is the most commonly used technique of ART. It involves retrieving mature eggs from a woman, fertilizing them with sperm in the laboratory, and implanting the embryos in the uterus 2 to 6 days after fertilization is confirmed.[19] This now-common procedure has given birth children to thousands of couples whose infertility would have left them childless only one generation ago.

The first IVF "test tube baby" was born in England in 1978. This birth was a historic moment marking the first time a human was ever conceived outside a mother's womb. The British doctors responsible for this breakthrough event, Drs. Robert Edwards and Patrick Steptoe, had labored for years trying to help women with blocked fallopian tubes, without success. They could surgically remove her eggs and fertilize them in the lab, yet they couldn't figure out why the embryos failed to develop into pregnancies once they were returned to the mother.

The turning point came when Drs. Steptoe and Edwards decided to transfer the embryo earlier, allowing it to divide only three times before placing it in the womb.[20] Today, a perfectly healthy and "normal" 24-year-old Louise Brown is the result.

Three years later, in 1981, Elizabeth Jordan Carr, America's first IVF baby, was born, and many more have followed her. The ASRM tells us that since that time, more than 45,000 babies have been born in the United States as a result of this medical technique.[21]

Today IVF is a standard treatment for infertility. But when Louise Brown and Elizabeth Carr were born, it was very controversial and raised innumerable moral issues. Arthur Caplan, from the Center for Bioethics at the University of Pennsylvania, remembers that many unanswered questions persisted at that time: "Were you going to have a child born who had birth defects? Were you going to have developmental abnormalities? Would something go wrong later in the life of that person? I think the terror was that, somehow, doing something in a dish was going to create a person that was less than healthy," he says.[22] Now, just a short quarter of a century later, IVF has become the starting point for treating almost every cause of infertility, allowing problems such as defective eggs, weak sperm, and abnormal chromosomes (once insurmountable obstacles) to be overcome.

To achieve pregnancy, six steps must be accomplished successfully:

1. Ovulation
2. Egg retrieval
3. Sperm retrieval and processing

Parentage Options with Artificial Insemination

Three different kinds of parentage can result from artificial insemination depending on a couple's type of infertility:

1. Artificial insemination of the mother with father's sperm

2. Artificial insemination of the mother with donor sperm

3. Artificial insemination of a surrogate mother with the father's sperm

4. Sperm and egg fertilization
5. Embryo transfer
6. Implantation.

The following sections will take a look at what you can expect each step of the way.

Step 1: Ovulation

The success of ART begins with a healthy egg. Some infertility programs will wait for the woman's natural cycle to produce an egg for harvesting, but most try to maximize a couple's chances of pregnancy by using a process called *superovulation:* prescribing fertility drugs to make multiple fertilizable eggs available at the time of the scheduled egg retrieval. Drugs commonly used for this purpose are the same ones used before insemination: injectable gonadotropins (Follistim, Gonal-F, Pergonal, Repronex) and human chorionic gonadotropin (hCG).

Generally, the woman begins taking ovulation-inducing drugs between the first and fifth days of her cycle to stimulate the development of multiple follicles. (Some medications are given through daily subcutaneous or intramuscular injections. In these cases, the partner or the woman herself may be taught how to administer the shot.)

The woman is monitored closely during this time. Blood hormonal levels are tested during the first week of stimulation, then daily. Ultrasound exams help the doctor watch the growth in size of ovarian follicles. The dosage and scheduling of the medications may be changed based on these findings. Cervical mucus monitoring also may be used to determine the exact time of ovulation. When the follicles reach maturity, usually after 7 to 10 days of medication, an hCG injection is administered to trigger egg maturation. In most cases, 35 to 36 hours later, the eggs will be ready for retrieval.

Step 2: Egg Retrieval

In IVF, mature eggs are removed from the ovaries to be fertilized outside the woman's body. The eggs (oocytes) can be retrieved from the ovarian follicles surgically in one of two ways, using either mild sedation or general or local anesthesia. The doctor may choose to make what's called a *transabdominal transfer* via laparoscopy. In this case, a catheter is guided through the abdomen through an incision near the naval. Two smaller incisions are made in the pubic hairline for egg

Who Uses IVF?

According to the American Society for Reproductive Medicine, fewer than 5 percent of infertile couples in treatment use IVF. Most commonly, the procedure is recommended for the following individuals:

- Women with blocked, severely damaged, or absent fallopian tubes
- Women with endometriosis
- Couples with infertility caused by male factor infertility
- Couples with long-term, unexplained infertility, unresponsive to other treatments[23]

retrieval instruments. The follicles are punctured with a thin needle inserted through the laparoscope. Fluid is withdrawn from each follicle. This fluid is then examined under a microscope for eggs.

Eggs are also retrieved through a less invasive and more popular process called a *transvaginal ultrasound-guided follicular aspiration*. In this case, an ultrasound probe is inserted into the woman's vagina. Using a needle guide attached to the probe, the doctor harvests the eggs by puncturing the follicles with a long, skinny needle. The fluid and eggs are then aspirated into the needle and withdrawn. The procedure takes less than 20 minutes.

Dr. Sills says that the number of eggs retrieved is influenced by the age of the woman. "In our practice," he says, "we are usually able to get around 12 or 13 eggs per patient. The older patient will have

IVF Without Stimulation Drugs

Powerful ovary-stimulating drugs have become a standard part of IVF. But according to a new British study out of King's College Hospital in London, the procedure can be made safer and almost as effective when doctors rely instead on a woman's natural menstrual cycle. In this study, 52 women went through three or four IVF treatment cycles based on their natural menstrual cycles. Their live birth rate was 32 percent, which compares favorably to the 34 percent success rate of women treated with drug-stimulated IVF. The researchers believe that the natural cycle IVF avoids the risk of ovarian hyperstimulation syndrome, greatly cuts the cost of treatment, and allows the couple to begin a second cycle immediately if the procedure fails. The researchers say that the best candidates for natural IVF are couples with unexplained infertility, women with fallopian tube problems, and women with regular menstrual cycles.[24]

fewer. Since the number of eggs naturally produced each month is usually just one, we can offer a substantial improvement in egg yield through controlled ovarian hyperstimulation and egg retrieval." Once the eggs are retrieved, they are immediately placed into culture medium and stored in an incubator.

In the future, the egg retrieval may be performed at an earlier stage through a process called *in vitro maturation*. This technique involves the intentional retrieval of oocytes before they are fully mature, with subsequent "growth"

> *The number of eggs retrieved is influenced by the age of the woman.*

in the laboratory. The goal is to reduce the amount of fertility drugs necessary to produce eggs and to decrease the number of eggs allowed to mature and thus the number of possible surplus embryos. Dr. Sills says this approach is still an experimental idea. "This is not yet considered mainstream medical practice," he says, "because we don't know with precision what cellular signaling processes are necessary to mature an egg. Despite the many advancements in in vitro embryo culture, we still haven't excelled over the in vivo model. If I have to pick between having an egg mature in the ovary or in the laboratory, I'd say let the egg mature in the body."

Step 3: Sperm Retrieval and Processing

On the day of the egg retrieval, the male partner will give a sperm sample through masturbation, or samples previously given and frozen will be thawed. The semen will undergo the standard analysis. Then it will be washed and perhaps challenged to "swim up" to obtain the healthiest sperm. Although you won't need to be involved in the sperm processing, in case you're interested in what happens, here's a technical rundown.

Sperm washing is a laboratory technique for separating sperm from semen, and motile sperm from nonmotile sperm. The ejaculate is placed in a culture medium, similar to the fluid found in the female reproductive tract, and it is then spun slowly in a centrifuge to separate the sperm from the seminal fluid. This is repeated two or three times. The concentrated sperm are then resuspended in solutions appropriate for the ART procedure, loaded into a syringe, and deposited into the uterus.

In the "sperm rise" or "swim-up" technique, semen or washed sperm are placed at the bottom of a tube of culture medium. The best sperm literally swim up into the top layer, where they are recovered and used for the ART procedure.

In some cases, the male is unable to obtain any healthy sperm in his ejaculate. In the past, this male factor problem meant a life without biological children. However, now medical procedures can be performed under appropriate anesthesia or sedation to extract sperm from parts of the male reproductive tract such as the epididymis, vas deferens, or testicle. Specifically, four procedures can recover sperm:

Microsurgical epididymal sperm aspiration (MESA). This is microsurgery to remove sperm from the epididymis.

> Sperm washing *is a laboratory technique for separating sperm from semen, and motile sperm from nonmotile sperm.*

Percutaneous epididymal sperm aspiration (PESA). A small needle is passed directly into the head of the epididymis, and fluid is aspirated.

Testes biopsy. A fragment of testicular tissue is extracted and examined under a microscope. The biopsy may be what's called "open," in which a small piece of testicular tissue is removed through a skin incision; this is called a *testicular sperm extraction* (TESE). Or, the biopsy may be performed using a spring-loaded needle that is inserted into the testicle; this technique is called a *testicular sperm aspiration* (TESA). Drs. Goldstein and Schlegel state that testes biopsy "is indicated in men who are azoospermic [having an absence of sperm in the ejaculate] with testes of normal size, normal consistency, palpable vasa deferentia, and normal serum FSH levels."[25]

Electroejaculation (EEJ). A high incidence of men with physical and neurological disorders (such as spinal cord injuries, multiple sclerosis, and spina bifida; and men after cancer treatment and retroperitoneal lymph node dissections) are infertile due to ejaculatory failure. Fortunately, the technology of electroejaculation has greatly improved the outlook for these men. Dr. Seaman says, "We don't understand exactly how electroejaculation works, but we do know that it can be very successful. To perform the procedure, an electric probe is placed inside the rectum against the prostate and seminal vesicles. This 'shocks' the sperm to be ejaculated out of the body." This can be a painful procedure and therefore is most often used in men who have no sensation in the rectum. Those who do have intact rectal sensation require general anesthesia. "Typically," says Dr. Seaman, "the sperm count and sperm quality after an electroejaculation are poor, but often good enough for an in vitro fertilization and sometimes even good enough for an insemination."

Electroejaculation has answered a prayer—three times over—for Louis and Kathi. When Louis was 19, his motorcycle was hit by a driver making a U-turn, and he was told he'd never walk again. "I'd only had my bike a month," Louis told a reporter from *Family Circle* magazine. "I didn't even know what the word *paraplegic* meant." He was also told that it was highly improbable that he would be able to father children. But after Louis married Kathi, they enrolled in the Miami Male Fertility Research Program, and after three attempts at electroejaculation and IVF, Kathi found herself pregnant with triplets.

"Couples have to really want to do this," says neuroscientist Nancy Brackett, Ph.D., who started the Miami program and now directs it. "We now have several dozen of them in treatment. What they all have in common is their optimism: They don't see obstacles; they see opportunities. Instead of resenting all they have to go through, they're grateful for the chance. I'm impressed every day with their deep commitment and gratified to see what fine parents they make once they do have children."[26]

Step 4: Sperm and Egg Fertilization

It's time to introduce the sperm to the eggs. For men with normal sperm counts, about 50,000 of the most motile sperm are mixed with each of the female's eggs. If a man has abnormally shaped sperm or a mild to moderately low sperm count or motility, as many as 5,000,000 sperm are mixed with each egg. The egg–sperm mixture is placed in an incubator for 2 to 12 hours after egg retrieval. A lot has to happen now: The egg's metabolism must be turned on, the sperm must find its way into the egg, a barrier must be erected to keep other sperm out, and the nuclei and chromosomes from the egg and sperm must be united inside the egg. The following day, the eggs are checked for fertilization. Generally, 80 percent of the mature eggs become fertilized at this stage.[27]

> *A*pproximately 30 percent of all ICSI cycles performed in the United States in 1998 resulted in a live birth, which is comparable to rates seen with traditional IVF.

Sometimes, during the fertilization phase, nothing happens. The eggs and sperm don't do what they're supposed to do—especially if the sperm are not healthy enough to find their way inside the egg. In the recent past, this occurrence would stop the IVF process, which would be chalked off as a failure. But as Daniel A. Dumesic, M.D., a reproductive endocrinologist at Mayo Clinic, Rochester, Minnesota, tells us, "In the last 3 or 4 years, we've seen some remarkable progress in our ability to treat infertile men. One of the keys in this treatment has been the use of intracytoplasmic sperm injection." Unlike other male factor treatments that emphasize increasing the quantity or quality of sperm, *intracytoplasmic*

When to Use Intracytoplasmic Sperm Injection (ICSI)

At the Seventh International Congress on Assisted Reproductive Technology and Advancements in Infertility Management, presenters reported that if normal morphology, as assessed by strict criteria in sperm, is less than 14 percent in a semen sample, IVF is advised. But if the morphology is less than 4 percent, ICSI is recommended.[29]

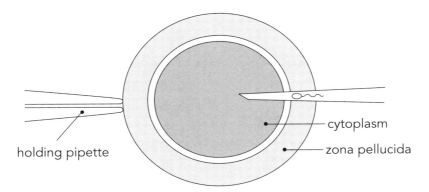

holding pipette

cytoplasm

zona pellucida

Figure 4.1—*Intracytoplasmic Sperm Injection (ICSI)*

sperm injection (ICSI) is a form of IVF in which a single sperm is injected directly into an egg to achieve fertilization. (See figure 4.1.)

This procedure increases the likelihood of fertilization when there are abnormalities in the number, quality, or function of the sperm that cause fertilization failure in the regular course of IVF. (In this procedure, the male needs to have only *one* quality sperm!) Fertilization occurs in 50 to 80 percent of injected eggs, but not all of those eggs develop properly—the fertilized egg may fail to divide, or the embryo may arrest at an early stage of development. Still, approximately 30 percent of all ICSI cycles performed in the United States in 1998 resulted in a live birth, which is comparable to rates seen with traditional IVF. Factors such as poor egg quality and advanced maternal age may result in lower rates of success, so younger couples may achieve more favorable results.[28] ICSI has largely replaced two other types of micromanipulation you may read about in older books: partial zona dissection (PZD) and subzonal insertion (SUZI) because it achieves higher overall fertilization rates.

The history of ICSI shows how successful research experiments are sometimes the result of a lucky accident. While performing a standard IVF, Gianpiero Palermo, M.D., of New York–Weill Cornell Medical Center, made a mistake. He explains, "I was placing sperm around the egg, underneath the shell, then accidentally I perforated

Miracle or Disaster?

A study conducted by Dr. David Page of the Whitehead Institute for Biomedical Research in Cambridge and Dr. Sherman Silber of the Infertility Center of St. Louis has shown that sons inherit the abnormal chromosome linked to male infertility. Dr. Page and colleagues tested 89 infertile men, of whom 12 were missing a fragment of the Y chromosome known as the AZFc region (a Y deletion mutation). The loss of the tiny piece appears to account for infertility for about 13 percent of men who produce little or no sperm, Dr. Page said. In their study, the authors examined four sons of three men who had a deletion in the AZFc region and had undergone ICSI. In all four cases, the sons had the same Y chromosome deletion.[30]

Dr. Jean Fourcroy, M.D., Ph.D., of the Uniformed Services University of Health Sciences in Bethesda, Maryland, says, "Modern medicine now allows men with genetically defective sperm to have biological children. Men with a missing Y chromosome, who before this time would never know the joy of holding a biological child in their arms, now can father children. But this joy is tempered with the knowledge that their progeny may have this same genetic gene mutation and will also be infertile. This is a questionable practice that can lead to a whole new population of men with built-in contraception."

the membrane of the egg. And then one sperm went inside. Ironically, I didn't pay much attention. I thought the egg would not survive the procedure. And I put a question mark to it because I thought it was going to die. But that was the only egg that fertilized. It finally was transferred to the patient, and this became the first ICSI baby."[31]

Step 5: Embryo Transfer (ET)

About 30 hours after fertilization, the sperm and egg have become a two-celled embryo. By 48 hours after fertilization, the embryo should have four cells, and by 60 hours, it should have divided into eight cells. Three or four embryos are usually transferred into the woman's uterus anywhere from the two-cell to the eight-cell stage (30 to 60 hours after fertilization). (See figure 4.2.)

In some cases, doctors are now using what is called *blastocyst transfer*. With this technique, the embryos are transferred to the uterine cavity at the 5-day rather than the usual 3-day stage. Ali Nasseri, M.D., co–medical director of Valley Hospital's Center for In Vitro Fertilization and Reproductive Endocrinology in Ridgewood, New Jersey, says, "This technique has several advantages. With blastocyst transfer, better quality embryos are transferred and the implantation

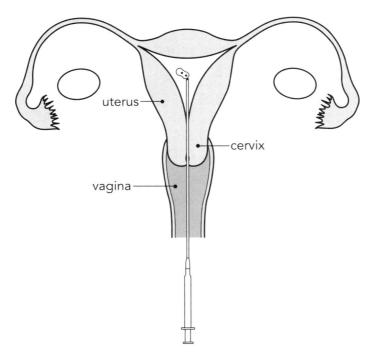

Figure 4.2—*IVF Transfer*

capability rate is greater. Also, at the 5-day stage, fewer embryos need to be transferred, decreasing the likelihood of multiple gestation."[32]

When the eggs are ready for transfer, the reproductive surgeon threads a thin plastic catheter through the woman's vagina, through the cervical canal, and into the uterus. He or she then transfers the fertilized embryos through the catheter similar to the process used with an IUI. This 10-minute outpatient procedure requires no anesthesia, but it can cause some discomfort and cramping. After the transfer, you'll lie still for about 1 to 2 hours. There may be some leakage of fluid, but it's no reason for panic. The embryos are tucked away and do not flow out with the excess fluid. Then you'll be told to go home and rest (lying down as much as possible) for the next 24 hours.

> *This 10-minute outpatient procedure requires no anesthesia, but it can cause some discomfort and cramping.*

There are some variations on the embryo transfer process that, in some rare cases, a doctor may choose in the hopes of improving chances of success. In the standard IVF procedure, the egg is placed into the woman's uterus. But in some IVF-like procedures, the embryo is placed inside the fallopian tube instead (of course, only when the woman has clear, open fallopian tubes). This is called *transuterine fallopian transfer* (TUFT) or *tubal embryo transfer* (TET). The transfer is made by threading a tube through the cervical canal and uterus and depositing the embryo into the fallopian tube. The process is meant to mimic the natural process of a fertilized embryo traveling down the tube and implanting in the uterus.

The IVF process can also be altered to change the timing of the egg transfer into the fallopian tube. In a method of assisted reproduction called *gamete intrafallopian transfer* (GIFT), after the egg is retrieved and sperm collected, the unfertilized gametes (the sex cells of the female and male—the eggs and sperm) are placed directly into the fallopian tube. The eggs are fertilized while in the fallopian tube and then move naturally down the tube into the uterus. This procedure involves major surgery that is not necessary in standard IVF.

Another procedure called *zygote intrafallopian transfer* (ZIFT) may also be used to allow the eggs and sperm to fertilize in the fallopian tube. In this procedure, a fertilized egg that has not yet divided (a zygote) is placed into a fallopian tube the day after removal. This procedure, too, requires a surgical procedure that is not required in IVF (see figure 4.3).

Step 6: Implantation

Once the gametes or embryos are tucked safely in your reproductive system, it's time to cross your fingers. It will take about 2 weeks to find out whether the IVF was a success. The embryo needs to implant itself into the uterine wall and continue to divide and develop. To help this process along, you will probably be given a hormone injection of hCG and may be placed on vaginal progesterone suppositories to keep the uterus receptive for the implantation.

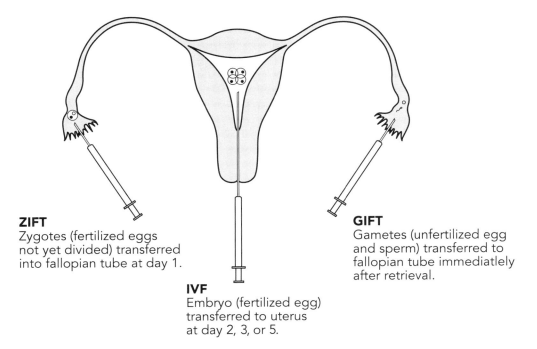

ZIFT
Zygotes (fertilized eggs not yet divided) transferred into fallopian tube at day 1.

GIFT
Gametes (unfertilized egg and sperm) transferred to fallopian tube immediatlely after retrieval.

IVF
Embryo (fertilized egg) transferred to uterus at day 2, 3, or 5.

Figure 4.3—*IVF, GIFT, ZIFT Comparison*

IVF Success Rates

You'll find that each part of the ART process has its own concerns and worries because failure can occur at any point. For example, let's take a hypothetical group of 30 women who start the ovulation stimulation process to begin IVF. Of this group, some may have the process stopped right in the beginning because not enough eggs are produced. Of the remaining women who undergo egg retrieval, some will have eggs that don't fertilize and divide. Of those who have embryo transfers, only a small group will achieve a clinical pregnancy. And of that small group, some will miscarry. Only a select few will have a live born infant. But all 30 begin with hope, and that's what makes so many willing to try again and again.

> *It will take about 2 weeks to find out whether the IVF was a success.*

Dr. Sills believes that the success of IVF has been made more dramatic by the media than it really is. "We should remember," he cautions, "that in nature when a man and a woman have intercourse at just the right time and everything is optimum, there is only a 20 percent chance that the woman will become pregnant. When it doesn't work naturally, the couple can shrug their shoulders and try again next month. But when the same outcome happens after you've spent $15,000 and you've come to the doctor's office for the last 8 days having sonograms and blood tests, and you've been giving yourself injections for the last 2 weeks, then it's a very different emotional reaction when you get that negative pregnancy result.

"I'd like to tell couples that IVF has a 90 percent success rate," he adds, "but that would not be honest. In the best of all possible worlds with a young female (under age 35), we're looking at a 55 to 65 percent pregnancy rate per transfer in IVF. If that were a grade on a college class, that would be an F. And the odds go down from there when age, male factor infertility, and other difficulties are factored in. The doctor must clearly explain the limits of current treatments, despite the wonderful advancements that have been made in the last decade, before a couple embarks on this journey."

Which Method Is Best?

The success of the different IVF techniques is comparable, but considerable differences exist among program techniques, patient backgrounds, and the way that success rates are measured. Some programs have more success with GIFT than with IVF. Because IVF, ZIFT, and GIFT haven't been compared in the same series of patients, it isn't possible to say that one technique yields a higher pregnancy rate than another. But by comparing the results of these procedures on different groups of women, some researchers have offered statistical data that you will find as you research IVF success rates—data that are often contradictory.

According to a study at Tel Aviv University in Israel, women who fail to get pregnant after repeated cycles of IVF and conventional intrauterine embryo transfer (ET) can benefit from ZIFT. In this study, 83 women, whose mean age was 35 and who had a minimum of four previous failed IVF-ET cycles, were randomized to undergo ZIFT or blastocyst transfer (BT), while a control group underwent a fifth ET. Pregnancy rates were 38 percent for the ZIFT group, 13 percent for the ET group, and 0 percent for the women who had BT.[34] Statistics published by the

> **No Greater Risk**
>
> Research shows that there is no higher risk of genetic abnormalities in a child conceived with ART.[33]

U.S. Centers for Disease Control and Prevention and the Society for Assisted Reproductive Technology agree. These statistics show that implantation in the fallopian tube, which is more risky and more costly, has a higher success rate for fertilization.[35] But still there is debate.

Steven Palter, M.D., assistant professor and clinic chief of reproductive medicine in the Department of Obstetrics and Gynecology at the Yale School of Medicine, has published a study that contradicts these findings. "Our study shows that there is no difference in implantation and pregnancy rates among women undergoing zygote intrafallopian transfer (ZIFT) and intrauterine embryo transfer (ET)," said Dr. Palter, who presented his findings at a meeting of the American Society for Reproductive Medicine. He said that he and his coauthor,

Antonia Habana, analyzed 24 studies, which included several randomized, controlled trials. The researchers reviewed 548 cycles, which is the number of IVF attempts; 514 egg retrievals, and 388 transfers into the uterus or fallopian tube. Each case was comparable in terms of mean age, the cause of the infertility, the protocol used, and the number of transfers. They found the implantation rate and pregnancy rates were not significantly different.[36]

So which method of embryo transfer is best for you? Your doctor will advise you based on your age, your medical and infertility history, as well as financial and personal factors. But according to one woman who endured six failed IVF procedures before she found success, the best judge of what will work best for you is your own awareness of your body. Her story is on page 168.

> **Stats on Live Births**
>
> Similar to rates achieved by fertile couples, 78 percent of IVF procedures that result in pregnancy ultimately lead to a live birth. Of that 78 percent, about 50 percent are singletons, 24 percent are twins, and 5 percent are triplets or more.[37]

Extra Embryos

After in vitro fertilization and embryo transfer, many couples are faced with an important decision: What to do with the surplus fertilized eggs that are not transferred back into the woman for implantation? Some couples donate their extra embryos to other infertile couples, and others offer them to the IVF team for research purposes. These are very personal and often difficult decisions that you and your spouse must consider carefully.

Most couples choose to have their extra embryos frozen for later use; this option is called *cryopreservation*. The eggs can then be thawed if an IVF fails and the couple wants to try again, or if they want to repeat the process at a later time to have more children. This process lowers the total cost of repeated IVF treatments, and it also allows the embryos to be transferred during a natural ovulation cycle when the woman's uterus is naturally ready for implantation.

Although frozen and then thawed embryos may sound too futuristic for some, the process has been proven to be safe based on both experiential evidence and research studies. In one study, for example, a team from the University of Bologna, Italy, announced the results of a follow-up study of children born from frozen eggs. They studied 11 pregnancies that resulted in 13 children. The gestational age at delivery was normal, and the 5-minute Apgar scores were reported in the normal range. Postnatal growth and development have been followed, and the researchers have concluded that oocyte freezing appears to be safe, giving rise to normal children.[38]

Michael Wilson, M.D., a reproductive physiologist of the Reproductive Resource Center of Greater Kansas City, explains how cryopreservation works. He says that the embryos are stored in liquid nitrogen at –384 degrees at various stages of development from a single cell to 100-cell blastocysts. They are kept in tiny straws that are about 6 inches long and 2 millimeters in diameter, designed specifically for holding frozen embryos. The straws hold between one and three embryos, suspended in about 2 cubic centimeters of a solution of saltwater with nutrients very similar to the medium found in a woman's uterus. Many straws holding several hundred embryos are contained within a squat, round, double-walled thermos that is wider at the base and narrower at the neck to minimize vaporizing of the liquid nitrogen when the container is opened. Each clinic sets its own price for this storage service, but the cost most typically falls between $100 and $250 a year.[39]

> **Eggs to Spare**
>
> Some clinics have programs called "egg sharing." In this case, the clinic pays for the woman's infertility treatment and medications, and she gives half of all retrieved eggs back to the clinic to be used as egg donations for women who cannot harvest their own.

WHAT'S NEXT?

If the IVF cycle fails, the couple has an important decision to make. They need to decide whether they should try again or not. Most are advised to try four IVF cycles before giving up if they can afford to both financially and emotionally. If they choose to try again, their first

Traci: Success After Six Cycles

Traci was just a few months short of her 30th birthday, and her husband was 31 years old when they married 5 years ago. At the time, neither expected to have any trouble starting a family. In fact, after being married only 3 months, they decided to give up the pill and have a baby. Three-and-a-half years later, they were still childless.

"After 6 months of trying with nothing happening," says Traci, "I found out I had a blocked tube from a congenital defect and a polyp on my uterus. I had the polyp removed and the tube repaired surgically, but even after doing Clomid with IUI and then Follistim/IUI, it still wasn't working."

So 2 years after they first began trying to have a baby, Traci and her husband decided to try IVF. But the IVF didn't work right away, either—in fact, five cycles failed. But Traci says that each failure taught them and their doctor something that helped make the sixth attempt successful. "I did a lot of reading, I got books and articles, I went online, and I learned as much as I could. I also learned about how my own body responded. I kept very careful records of things like my temperature, my cervical fluid, every ultrasound, and how many follicles and what size and on what side. I wrote down all my hormone levels every time they were tested. I used this information to figure out what would work best for me. For example, I learned that the higher the estrogen level on the day of the trigger shot, the better results I got. When the estrogen level was at 150, I got bad results, so I knew the levels had to be pushed higher. When I was up to 200, I got pregnant."

Traci did a 3-day transfer on the first IVF because she didn't have enough quality embryos to do a blastocyst transfer on day 5. But the next four times, she did the 5-day transfers. "These gave me two chemical pregnancies [the hormonal levels indicate that pregnancy has occurred, but shortly afterward it fails] and one miscarriage," says Traci. "This was all so incredibly cruel, and yet at the same time, I still had hope because my doctor said that having chemical pregnancies is an extremely good indicator of future success." These failures sent Traci back for more diagnostic testing looking for uterine abnormalities, infection, or even toxicology problems. "I'm an organic chemist in the pharmaceutical industry, and I work with chemicals all the time," says Traci, "so we even checked to see if my job had anything to do with my infertility, but everything seemed fine."

On the final IVF, Traci's doctor decided to go back to a 3-day transfer so he could transfer more embryos and boost the odds. He transferred a total of five (a lot for a 33-year-old woman—the usual number is three embryos), and one implanted and developed into a successful pregnancy. Traci now has a beautiful 1-year-old daughter.

For anyone, six is a lot of IVF cycles to go through. Traci knows that with each negative result, it gets harder to hear the bad news and harder to try again. "Every time it doesn't work, there's a grieving process that you have to go through," she says. "You have to let yourself go through that. People would say things like, 'God has something he wants you to learn,' and I would think, 'I've learned enough!' But I found that if I let myself mourn what might have been, I could put those feelings to rest, take a deep breath, and plunge in again.

"The IVF cycles are not that hard to go through physically, but the emotional and financial aspects can be daunting," admits Traci. "We were lucky enough to have insurance coverage, so for us the decision to keep trying was easy. However, I have many friends who have paid for cycles out of their own pockets. They give up a lot in order to afford the treatments. Some have attained their dreams; others haven't. IVF is not a guaranteed process, but it's often the best hope for infertile couples who want their own biological child.

"My husband and I joke about 'the normals'—those people that can get pregnant just by having sex," she says. "Wouldn't it be nice if it were that easy for us? But when I look at my daughter, I know it was all worth it. All the heartache and tribulations seem so far away now. I'm already making plans to do it again."

question is, "When?" The answer, according to Dr. Sills, usually depends on the female's age.

According to data presented at the 1998 Ovulation Induction Conference in Bologna, Italy, there may be some slight benefit to delaying a second IVF treatment more than 40 days. But Dr. Sills and colleagues from Cornell showed in this presentation that while the long-term consequences of repeated IVF cycles with minimum rest intervals are unknown, rapid sequential ovarian stimulation does not appear to affect ovarian response, egg production, or pregnancy rate.

"I tell patients," says Dr. Sills, "that it takes more than just 1 month to build an egg. The events that foreshadow recruitment of the follicles may have been going on for 2 or 3 months before the IVF cycle, so if you do rapid, sequential IVF cycles, you have to wonder if there could be some deleterious, cumulative effect on the eggs for a subsequent cycle. But, of course, couples who are in their 40s don't want to take off 3 months in between cycles, so it is an impossible decision for them. Waiting might optimize egg quality, but while they're waiting, the clock is ticking and they may pass another birthday. It has to be individualized because the fact is that we don't know with much certainty how long a couple should wait between IVF cycles.

"In most centers," Dr. Sills continues, "the women are premedicated in the month before the scheduled cycles. That means if you wanted to do a cycle in June, on day 21 of your May menstrual cycle,

The Order of Events

Although each and every infertility case must be individually treated based on unique factors, in general, many couples progress through the process in this order:

1. Fertility drugs
2. Insemination
3. IVF or GIFT

you would begin to prepare for the June IVF. If the June cycle fails and you wanted to repeat IVF as soon as possible, you would still have to wait until cycle day 21 of your June period to start preparing for a July IVF. However, it may not be possible to work this so quickly, and the patient may find herself waiting for a July period."

Sometimes your body will mandate a longer waiting phase between IVF attempts. "If a woman comes back to prepare for another cycle and we find that she has some residual cysts in her ovaries from the previous failed cycle," cautions Dr. Sills, "she should not start again until they resolve and the ovaries are clear again—a process that could be complete within a month, but sometimes birth control pills are used to hasten the clearance of such cysts."

TWENTY-FOUR WAYS TO MAKE A BABY

This chapter has covered a number of assisted reproduction technology options. They are not all inclusive; new, improved, and simply different techniques are being explored by reproductive specialists all over the world on any given day. The methods described here give you a good overview of the most commonly used techniques. According to the information gathered here, there are at least 24 ways to make a baby through ART:

1. Artificial insemination—of mother with father's sperm
2. Artificial insemination—of mother with donor sperm
3. Artificial insemination—intrauterine
4. Artificial insemination—intracervical
5. Artificial insemination—intratubal
6. IVF—using egg and sperm of parents
7. IVF—with superovulation
8. IVF—with intracytoplasmic sperm injection (ICSI)
9. IVF—with in vitro maturation
10. IVF—with frozen embryos
11. IVF—with egg donor

12. IVF—with sperm donor
13. IVF—with egg and sperm donor
14. IVF—with assisted hatching
15. IVF—with fragment removal
16. IVF—with testicular sperm aspiration (TESA) or testicular sperm extraction (TESE)
17. IVF—with microsurgical epididymal sperm aspiration (MESA)
18. IVF—with percutaneous epididymal sperm aspiration (PESA)
19. IVF—with electroejaculation (EEJ)
20. IVF—with 3-day embryo transfer
21. IVF—with 5-day embryo transfer
22. IVF—with transuterine fallopian transfer (TUFT) or tubal embryo transfer (TET)
23. Gamete intrafallopian transfer (GIFT)
24. Zygote intrafallopian transfer (ZIFT)

These numbers are only the beginning. They do not count the various combinations of GIFT and ZIFT with many of the IVF procedures, and they do not include the surrogate options that will be discussed in the next chapter. But they do show that the field of assisted reproductive technology is growing in its capability to offer the infertile couple a child of their own.

ART is not an easy process. Some call it grueling; others say it is pure hell. No doubt it is emotionally draining as you hold your breath waiting to see whether there are enough eggs to harvest, whether the eggs fertilize, then whether and how many eggs implant resulting in pregnancy, and yet again whether the embryo will develop to term or will abort. All the while you know the odds are against you. So where is the upside? The upside is in the hope that these techniques offer. The desire to have a biological child is so deep and strong in some couples that the inconvenience of going through hell is no obstacle.

Infertility Options
Donor Eggs/Sperm, Surrogate Parenting, Adoption, and Nonparenting

AT SOME POINT, some infertile couples realize that, despite the most advanced methods of assisted reproduction technology and their own best efforts, they cannot conceive and carry a child of their own. If you are at this point, you need to ask yourself, "If I can't go down the fertility road any longer, is there a branch off this road that I would like to take?" Possible alternate routes discussed in this chapter include donor gametes, surrogate parenting, adoption, and nonparenting. Not one of these options is better than the other. Each one offers benefits and rewards for some couples while being completely inappropriate or unacceptable for others. To help you make an informed decision about your next step, this chapter gives you a brief overview of each possibility, some expert input, anecdotal stories, and resources for more information.

DONOR GAMETES

Sometimes there is no medical cure for eggs that won't fertilize. Sometimes the male's lack of quality sperm cannot be corrected or bypassed.

In years past, that was the end of the story for these couples—there would be no pregnancy and no genetic link to a child of their own. Today, there is renewed hope in egg and sperm donations—the medical substitution of the egg or sperm of the intended parents with that of a donor.

When considering donor insemination, only the couple involved knows what's right for them. Dr. Eric Scott Sills, who is director of oocyte donation at Georgia Reproductive Specialists in Atlanta, says, "It's important for the couple to consider what's most important to them. They need to ask, 'Is it to have a baby together? Or, to have a baby that is genetically ours?' There is a big difference between the two. If a couple wants the opportunity to share their love with a baby and nurture that child as parental figures, then adoption, for example, could fulfill that goal with limited medical intervention. But if the most important thing is to have a child with a genetic link, but the age or quality of the woman's eggs won't allow that to happen, we can medically substitute the egg of a younger woman and change her pregnancy success rate through IVF from somewhere around 1 percent up to nearly 60 percent.

> When considering donor insemination, only the couple involved knows what's right for them.

"Donor egg babies have been around since 1983," Dr. Sills explains. "We have continued to make refinements in this technique since then, so it is definitely within a couple's grasp to do this if necessary. The only caveat in this arrangement is the fact that the woman will not have a genetic connection to the child. But this is a very personal decision, and I like to have couples talk about it very carefully before they decide. If this is indeed something they want, then donor oocyte with IVF would be something that would have a relatively high yield in terms of pregnancy success rate."

The numbers are especially encouraging for women over 40. The most recent report from the United States National In Vitro Fertilization Embryo Transfer Registry indicate that 22 percent of the embryo transfers following IVF of donated oocytes resulted in live births, regardless of the woman's age. But a woman over 42 who undergoes IVF using her own oocytes has only a 4 percent chance of having a live birth per embryo transfer.[1]

The same promise of hope can be given to couples in which the male cannot produce enough quality sperm to fertilize an egg. By using sperm donation, his wife's egg can be fertilized through insemination or IVF. She can carry a fetus through the pregnancy and deliver a child that is genetically her own.

Finding the Right Donor

If you decide that using donor gametes is right for you, you will then begin the quest to find quality eggs or sperm. Administrators of most legitimate donor programs insist that donors be under 35, tattoo- and piercing-free, healthy, and, of course, fertile. After they make the first cut,

> *Twenty-two percent of the embryo transfers following IVF of donated oocytes resulted in live births, regardless of the woman's age.*

donors are subjected to genetic screening, psychological testing, and questions about their education and personal life. They are questioned about their sexual history and tested for communicable diseases. Some programs even do a criminal background check. However, not all donor programs follow these guidelines. Unless you use donor sperm or eggs obtained from a medically endorsed source, you have no way of knowing what you're getting. It is very difficult to check on the histories obtained from prospective donors, even if this were ethically correct.

Anonymous Donors

The growth of online donor sources has made it both easier and harder to find quality eggs and sperms—easier because of the greater number (and thus variety) to choose from, harder because that large number can make your search overwhelming and possibly include some con artists. Web sites such www.fertilityoptions.com and www.eggdonor.com are pioneering the business of producing online classified ads for egg and sperm donors.

"The Internet absolutely has increased the social acceptability of using egg donors," says Wendy Somers, director and founder of Creating Families (www.creatingfamilies.com). Doctors and clinics are still necessary for medical testing, performing egg implantation, administering drugs, and counseling patients. "But now you can choose from 500 donors nationwide instead of just 19 in your area," says Somers, whose site invites would-be parents to click on preferences for race, religion, college degrees, and hair and eye color.

Following this trend, the Atlanta-based Xytex, one of the largest sperm banks in the United States, allows men to submit all-about-me essays. The program has expanded to include photos and video interviews. Registered patients can see some of these online.[2]

> *One site invites would-be parents to click on preferences for race, religion, college degrees, and hair and eye color.*

Thanks to the Internet and the growing social acceptance of donor pregnancies, you no longer have to go into anonymous donor ART blindly, but you do have to be very careful. There are a lot of unscrupulous people out there who are willing to take advantage of your vulnerability to make a fast buck. Some people will promote themselves as donors without any real intentions of following through; others make offers to several people at once, take the money, and run. And it's certainly not unheard of for anonymous online donors to lie about their medical history. When this happens, you face the possibility of contracting viral infections such as hepatitis or AIDS. You also have no assurance about the quality of the sperm or egg and can't even be sure whether the medical report or sperm sample you get really belongs to the person you've contracted with. Unfortunately, one has to rely on the program's integrity and give up some control over the process.

The Cost of Anonymous Donor Eggs and Sperm

Men and women who donate their gametes are paid for the service. The compensation from above-board egg donation programs in New York hovers around $5,000. It's a hefty sum when compared to the

$50 sperm donors earn, though not so hefty when you consider the month of doctors appointments, physical and psychological tests, and drug taking that donors have to undergo, not to mention the fact that some believe that the drugs involved could increase the risk of ovarian cancer and other medical complications.[3]

In addition to the compensation fee, if you use a donor company to locate a donor, you will also pay legal and administrative fees. One online, and seemingly reputable, company advises clients up-front about all costs. For egg donors the cost includes the counselor's fee (covers screening, counseling, matching, and support), the company's retainer fee (covers administration, coordination, and advertising costs), legal/contract fees (covers contracts, independent legal representation for the recipient couple), the egg donor's fee, the egg donor's legal counsel, and an insurance policy that covers egg donor and egg recipient.

> *In addition to the compensation fee, if you use a donor company to locate a donor, you will also pay legal and administrative fees.*

The total for these expenses comes to $8,450. But these fees do not include any of the standard medical costs for insemination or IVF. Under some circumstances they may be covered by insurance if your policy covers infertility treatment, but most often the payment comes out of your pocket. The final cost ranges between $15,000 and $20,000.

An Ethical Issue

Although most agree that it's reasonable to compensate donors, something about selling eggs and sperm bothers a lot of people. In some cases, these vital components of creation become commodities, with the more "desirable" ones going for whopping fees. In 1999, a couple advertised in a number of Ivy League college newspapers that they would pay $50,000 for an egg from a tall, athletic, top college student with high College Board test scores. Later that same year, longtime fashion photographer, Ron Harris, offered models as egg donors to the highest bidders at an Internet auction geared to parents willing to pay up to $150,000 in hopes of having a beautiful child.[4] This concern hit the headlines again in 2000 when a couple placed a half-page ad in Stanford University's student newspaper offering $100,000 for the eggs of a bright, young, white athlete. This is all perfectly legal because federal law forbids the trafficking of human organs but not sperm or eggs. Still, mainstream infertility groups such as the American Society of Reproductive Medicine (ASRM) and RESOLVE feel the idea of asking high prices for extra-nice genes screams of unethical behavior.[5]

Nonanonymous Donors or Directed Donation

To avoid being scammed, many couples rely on anonymous sperm or oocyte donation programs recommended by their physician or a representative of a fertility clinic. Others keep control over the process by using the eggs or sperm from people they know and trust. This was the case for Susan when she and her husband, Mike, decided to give donor IVF a try.

Susan and Mike married in 1995 when she was 26 and he was 27. Less than a year later, this young couple decided to start their family, and 5 years later they finally have a wonderful baby boy to hold in their arms—but it wasn't easy. When Susan wasn't getting pregnant month after month, they realized that something was wrong and went to Susan's obstetrician for basic fertility testing. The doctor found no reason for the fertility difficulty but gave Susan a prescription for Clomid and then tried two inseminations. Both failed. Susan and her husband then moved on to a reproductive endocrinologist (RE).

"With this new doctor," remembers Susan, "I did three full in vitro cycles. Each time I responded well to the injectables, the eggs looked good, and they fertilized fine. We would transfer three or four embryos. The remaining embryos always fizzled out by day 5, so we never had any left over to freeze. Then 2 weeks later we would get the call that our cycle had failed." Susan still had no reason for her infertility, but clearly there was a problem. The doctor mentioned the option of using donor eggs.

Susan says she was not ready to give up on herself just yet, so she went to a new RE and tried two more cycles of IVF. Both of those were canceled just before the retrieval time because of poor stimulation by the medication. Again, the doctor suggested that the problem may be with the quality of the eggs and asked Susan to think about using donor eggs. "This is a hard decision to make," says Susan. "I grew up assuming I would grow up and have a family. I never thought that wouldn't happen for me. Even when I was having problems getting pregnant, I thought everything would eventually work out. But then comes a moment in time when the doctors tell you that you're wasting your time and money, and you realize that things aren't going to be just like you planned." Mike did not want to adopt, and he and Susan both worried about using anonymous donor eggs, so they just didn't know what to do next. Then the phone rang one night, and things fell into place.

"My cousin, who knew we had been trying for awhile, had heard from her mother (who heard from my mother) that our last IVF attempt had once again failed, so she called one night and offered to be the egg donor," says Susan with a smile. "I would never have asked her to do this, but I just felt so happy that she would do this for me. I was so relieved that my child would have family genes, and I would know everything about the medical and personal background."

Shortly afterward, Susan's 25-year-old single cousin began the donor process. She went for a medical and psychological exam; she took the injectable medications (just like a woman preparing for IVF), and then went in for the egg retrieval process. At the same time, Susan, too, began taking fertility medication by injection to suppress her ovaries so they wouldn't make any eggs. She also wore estrogen patches to prepare her uterus to receive the fertilized egg. When her cousin was ready to donate her eggs, Susan began getting shots of progesterone and taking medrol and doxycycline. On the day of the scheduled egg retrieval, Susan's

> *When her cousin was ready to donate her eggs, Susan began getting shots of progesterone and taking medrol and doxycycline.*

husband donated his sperm, and her cousin went into the clinic to have the egg retrieval performed. Three days later, when eggs had fertilized and divided, Susan went into the clinic to have the embryos transferred into her uterus. Then, with all fingers crossed, they all waited. (The worst part!)

Susan's cousin had recovery symptoms typical of woman who has IVF: a bit of bloating, cramping, and tenderness in the abdominal area. Susan felt fine physically after the embryos were implanted and was very optimistic that this was something that would finally work. But then 2 weeks later, Susan got her period; the donor transfer had failed. "We were all so disappointed, and I was truly crushed. It's so hard to try something new, get your hopes up, and then fail again," says Susan.

But persistent in hope, 2 months later, Susan repeated the transfer process with embryos that had been frozen after the first try—and it worked! Now Susan and Mike have a toddler running around their home. "I think of my son as 100 percent my own," Susan says. "I became emotionally attached to my baby when he was inside of me growing. And I think that being able to carry him and have the experience of pregnancy and labor was a big help."

Since that time, most of Susan's worries have eased. "During my pregnancy, I often wondered how my cousin and her family would react to my child and how they would feel once he was born; it worried me a little. I know that they feel closer to my son than they do to my brother's children, and I often wondered if it was going to bother me. But then my mom told me something that has helped me a lot. She said, 'There can never be too many people that love a child,' and that is something I always try to remember."

Susan's only concern now is how she will tell her son about all this, but that's down the road at another time. Right now, Susan is 6 months pregnant with twins, again using her cousin as a donor. She and Mike are thrilled that they will have two more children through the miracle of assisted reproductive technology.

SURROGATE PARENTING

Sometimes a woman simply cannot or should not conceive or carry a baby to term. She may not produce eggs; she may have eggs that will not fertilize; she may be afraid of passing on a genetic defect; she may have a medical condition that makes pregnancy inadvisable; she may have had a hysterectomy. In these cases, the only way to have a genetic offspring is to have another woman carry and give birth to her child—a surrogate mother arrangement. This option that seemed like science fiction not so long ago is now a viable alternative that many couples give serious consideration.

As with all forms of assisted reproduction, this choice requires a lot of thought, preparation, and guidance. This section will give you an overview of some of the basics: the types of surrogacy, the benefits, the risks, methods of finding a surrogate, the cost, and legal considerations. With these facts in hand, you'll have a good idea whether this approach is something you'd like to investigate further.

> *This option that seemed like science fiction not so long ago is now a viable alternative that many couples give serious consideration.*

Types of Surrogacy

There are three basic types of surrogacy:

Gestational surrogacy. A surrogate parenting arrangement in which an egg is retrieved from the wife of the intended couple, combined with her husband's sperm, and the resulting embryo is implanted in the surrogate. The child is not genetically related to the surrogate, and in many states the couple's names go on the original birth certificate.

Traditional surrogacy. A surrogate parenting arrangement in which the surrogate is artificially inseminated with the sperm from the husband of the intended couple. The child is genetically related to the surrogate and the intended father. The wife of the intended couple adopts the child.

Donor surrogacy. A surrogate parenting arrangement in which an embryo created in vitro with the genetic material of one of the intended parents (mother or father) and a donor egg or sperm is transferred to the surrogate. This child is genetically related to the intended parent who contributed the egg or sperm and the donor. It is not related to the surrogate. The intended parent who did not contribute egg or sperm will adopt the child after birth.

The Benefits of Surrogacy

Jimmy Shrybman of the Shrybman Law Offices in Maryland has practiced exclusively in child-related law and family expansion options since 1977 (www.surrogacy-solutions.com). His law firm as well as his adoption and surrogacy agency have handled hundreds of family cases. Over the years, Shrybman says he has noticed a reversal of interest. "When we first started, we were doing lots of private, domestic adoptions and some international adoptions; this was about 90 percent of our business. Today the numbers have flipped; now we do mostly surrogacies. When couples get beat up by all the disappointments and physical and emotional exhaustion that go with infertility treatments, those who are repeatedly unsuccessful will finally get to a point where they begin to look around at other options. The first place they look is at adoption. But this is not an easy or simple choice."

Being involved in both adoption and surrogacy cases, Shrybman feels he has an objective view of the pros and cons of each and understands why more and more couples are choosing surrogacy over adoption. "Adoption, especially a private domestic adoption, is often fraught with more risk and more disappointment than surrogate arrangements," he says. "There are thousands of stories about birth mothers who change their minds, or who disappear just before the birth, or who work with multiple couples at the same time, or who put the fetus at risk with substance abuse. There are the stories about birth fathers who won't sign papers or who show up at the last minute and decide they want the baby. Even after the baby is born and sent home with the adoptive couple, most states allow the birth mother a period of time in which to change her mind. These emotional risks, coupled with the financial risk involved in paying the birth mother's medical, legal, psychological, living, and personal expenses without any guarantee, bring many couples to see surrogacy as a safer emotional and financial investment."

When comparing the pros and cons of adoption and surrogacy, Shrybman reminds his clients that parents and surrogates enter surrogacy relationships for different reasons and from different legal positions than people in adoptive situations.

> *The genetic link that makes surrogacy desirable for many couples also provides them legal advantages not available in adoption.*

Surrogacy is essentially a contract for a service. The surrogate's reasons for becoming pregnant are to help the would-be parents become parents and to help her own family and herself with the compensation she earns for her services. The genetic link that makes surrogacy desirable for many couples also provides them legal advantages not available in adoption.

The Risks of Surrogacy

According to Shrybman, the biggest risk choosing surrogacy is medical, not legal or social. Like all assisted reproductions, there is a risk that conception will not occur. The insemination or IVF may fail, and the couple may then begin the infertility treatments with the surrogate that they have probably been through themselves. Also, like all pregnancies, there is the risk that the surrogate will miscarry, have a premature birth, or have prenatal problems that require special care. All the risks of any pregnancy accompany a surrogate pregnancy.

Couples always fear that the surrogate will change her mind and decide to fight them legally for custody of the child that she delivered. That fear is generally unfounded. Of the 2,000 or so births to surrogates in this country, a woman has refused to relinquish the child less than 1 percent of the time.[6] "Adoption is a win-lose situation in which either the birth mother suffers a loss and the adoptive parents walk away the winners, or the birth parent keeps the baby and the prospective adoptive parents end up empty-handed.

"But surrogacy is a win-win situation," says Shrybman. "The surrogate mother gets pregnant for the sole purpose of giving the child away and in some cases earning some money. She achieves her purpose only if the surrogate contract is carried out. The surrogate's husband (if there is one) already has kids and sure doesn't want to keep this one with another man's genes. And in the end, legally, the surrogate mother has claim to only half the child at best and would need to engage in an expensive and drawn-out legal custody battle where historically the child ends up with the intended parents. Change of mind doesn't make sense in a surrogacy arrangement."

The Controversial Side of Surrogacy

Although surrogacy is more attractive to some couples than adoption, the idea of surrogacy is still a controversial issue. On a moral, ethical, and religious level, many people are strongly against this form of reproduction. Some feel that this commercial arrangement reduces surrogates to the position of paid baby carriers. There is also concern that this is a form of infertility treatment available only to the rich. In addition, some worry that surrogate arrangements allow for "unnatural" births, such as the case of the mother who carried a triplet pregnancy conceived via IVF with her daughter's eggs and her son-in-law's sperm. She ended up giving birth to her own grandchildren! Of course, there was a time when any form of assisted reproduction was blasted as "unnatural," so the idea of surrogacy may just need more time to become fully accepted.

Finding a Surrogate

There are several ways to find a surrogate mother. Some couples find a family member or a friend who is willing to give the gift of a child to the infertile couple. This option became especially popular when Phoebe on the TV show *Friends* became a surrogate mother of triplets for her brother. This was the first time the option of surrogacy as a positive choice became part of our popular culture.

You can also select a surrogate through a surrogate agency. In this arrangement, the process is a lot like hiring an employee. You interview prospective candidates. You look over their background and experience. You question their motives and goals. You await the results of medical and psychological screenings. In the end, *you* decide who will carry your baby.

The typical surrogate is a woman in her mid-20s to early 30s, working, married, and the mother of her own children. When Shrybman interviews prospective surrogates, he looks for these characteristics:

- She already has children. The experience of giving birth for the first time is an overwhelming physical, emotional, life-changing event. That's not the kind of thing that should happen when giving birth as a surrogate.

- Her former pregnancies have been easy, and she likes being pregnant.

- She is the kind of person who wants to do something good for somebody.

- She is happy with her life.

- She really wants the money. She may have many altruistic reasons for wanting to do this, but like with any job, the money is important. And she wants the money for something major—not just to pay today's bills. She wants to earn the money for a down payment on a house. She wants to send her own child to a good college. She herself wants to go back to school and earn a degree.

Cost of Surrogacy

The cost of surrogacy depends on many factors. If your sister is your surrogate and is not taking any fee for this service and you are using artificial insemination, your cost will be far less than the couple who goes to an agency and selects an anonymous surrogate and uses an IVF procedure. The fees involved generally cover expenses such as the following:

Legal expenses. These include contract preparation, final preparation of the adoption decree, and any other legal work necessary to ensure that an accurate birth certificate and a decree of adoption and/or termination of parental rights are successful obtained.

Medical expenses. These include physical exams and sperm count of the father, insemination/embryo transfer, prenatal, delivery, and postpartum care for the surrogate. These costs will vary depending on the intended parents' and surrogate's health insurance policy, the type of assisted reproduction used (insemination or IVF), and the number of cycles necessary to achieve pregnancy.

Psychological fees. These are the costs for the psychological evaluation and testing for the surrogate.

Surrogate fee. This is the price the surrogate charges for this service. It runs anywhere from $0 to $20,000.

Surrogate Mothers, Inc., in Indiana, advises their intended couples that approximate expenses can be as little as $15,000 (if the surrogate is not charging any fee and has her own insurance) or as much as $50,000 (if she is asking $20,000 and does not have insurance). The average total cost is around $37,000.[7]

The Legal Side of Surrogate Parenting

Before you decide you want to pursue a surrogate pregnancy, you'll first need to check out the laws in your state. Not all states allow surrogate arrangements; New Jersey and New York, for example, do not. Other states allow surrogacy with insemination but not IVF. Others construe surrogacy as a form of adoption, and because you cannot pay compensation to a birth mother in an adoption, you cannot pay a surrogate, and so your pool of potential surrogates is limited. If you find that your state's laws make surrogacy impossible or difficult, you can make the arrangement in another state that is surrogate-friendly and where non-residents can adopt (so the intended mother can adopt her husband's biological child). You can start your exploration of state laws by visiting the Web site of the American Surrogacy Center, Inc. (TASC), at www.surrogacy.com and clicking the link for legal information. Here you will find an up-to-date review of the laws on surrogacy in each state.

If you find that your state's laws make surrogacy impossible or difficult, you can make the arrangement in another state that is surrogate-friendly and where non-residents can adopt.

A Surrogate Success Story

Brenda and Doane are attorneys from Washington, D.C., who married in their mid-30s and tried to start their family right away. It wasn't long before Brenda learned that she had poor quality eggs due to age-related factors. Although she tried the fertility drug Clomid to improve ovulation, this treatment was abandoned when she had an allergic reaction that affected her eyesight. This was when Brenda and Doane decided that they did not want to get further involved with infertility treatments.

"We knew from the start that we didn't want to try IVF," says Brenda. "The doctor was pessimistic that it would work with my eggs, and it was just too expensive to attempt against the odds. Also, for religious reasons my husband didn't want to risk having to use selective reduction on excess embryos, and we knew there were health risks in carrying multiple fetuses. So the whole thing just wasn't the right choice for us."

Brenda and Doane had just about given up trying to have their own child as they reached 40 and were starting to talk about adoption when a fellow lawyer told them that he and his wife where having a baby through surrogacy. The experience was so positive for this couple that Brenda and Doane decided to go the same route. "We contacted a surrogate attorney who gave us some profiles to look through. The women who apply to be surrogates fill out a five-page questionnaire that helps you get to know them. We found a woman who was just perfect for us. She was fair-skinned like my side of the family. She had a master's degree and a good job. She was divorced and had one child. We were very happy to learn that she was of my husband's religion and would not want to abort a child if there was a medical problem. This is how we felt about abortion if I had been able to get pregnant myself, so we certainly felt the same way about a baby conceived by a surrogate. We knew this was a good match."

Finding the right surrogate was key for Brenda and Doane. "Some of the woman we looked into," remembers Brenda, "seemed to have a lot of instability in their lives, and this worried us. One admitted using cocaine. Another submitted a picture of herself enjoying a wine cooler. These things just gave us a bad feeling. We knew we would not have total control over how a woman took care of herself and the baby during the pregnancy, so we kept looking until we found someone who made us feel really comfortable."

After making their choice and drawing up the necessary legal contracts, Brenda and Doane were ready to begin the surrogacy process. Their surrogate, however, hit a slight fertility snag. After going off her birth control method, she did not again begin to ovulate. The fertility doctor recommended a cycle of fertility drug injections to get the ovaries functioning again.

> *When the surrogate delivered the baby, Brenda was right beside her.*

When the surrogate was ready, she was inseminated with Doane's sperm. Unfortunately, the first try was a failure. But, on the second try the following month, she became pregnant and their joint pregnancy began. "We kept in touch a lot throughout the pregnancy by e-mail," says Brenda. "And I went to several of the prenatal medical visits with her. The more I got to know her, the more I liked her and felt confident that this was the right choice for us."

When the surrogate delivered the baby, Brenda was right beside her. "Because her first child was born by cesarean section, the doctor suggested the same form of delivery this time, and so I was able to meet her at the hospital at the scheduled time and be present for the birth. (My husband was a little squeamish, and so he opted to wait outside.) As soon as he was born, the nurse placed my son in my arms," remembers Brenda, still moved to tears by the memory. "I was the first to hold him, and it was absolutely wonderful!"

Although some couples choose to break all ties with the surrogate at the time of birth, Brenda, Doane, and their surrogate have chosen to have an ongoing relationship. The surrogate held the baby and fed him his bottle during the 2 days they were in the hospital. Now that the baby is 1 month old, Brenda and the surrogate still talk occasionally, and Brenda sends her pictures by mail. Brenda says she will invite

---

Resource Referrals

For more information about donors and surrogate parenting, check out these Web sites:

Infertility Resources
www.ihr.com/infertility

Families 2000
www.families2000.com

The American Surrogacy Center
www.surrogacy.com

Organization of Parents Through Surrogacy
www.opts.addr.com/opts.htm

Surrogate Alternatives, Inc.
www.surrogatealternatives.net

Surrogate Mothers Online
www.surromomsonline.com

Surrogate Mothers, Inc.
www.surrogatemothers.com

the surrogate to the christening but expects that in time their contact will be less and less frequent.

"It has been good for all of us this way," Brenda says. "Although our surrogate is not looking to be a second mother to my son, and we do have separate lives, I want her to know how he's doing."

Brenda has had no problem bonding with this child with whom she has no genetic link. "When he's hungry, I'm the one holding him, and that's what matters most to me," she says. "I love when he looks so intently at my face like he's studying me. I know this is an unusual way to have a baby and not everyone is comfortable with our choice, but for us it could not have been better. Of course, it would be wonderful if we could have a child who was biologically both of ours. It would be thrilling to look into the baby's face and say, 'He has a nose just like my grandfather.' But since we can't have that, this certainly is the next best thing. He carries Doane's family's genes, and for that I'm happy."

ADOPTION

If you decide that parenting a child is more important to you than conceiving and bearing a child or having your own biological child, you may decide to adopt. It's very possible that a child is out there who needs parents just as much as you need a child. But it's difficult to take that first step. If the idea of the adoption process seems overwhelming to you, consider that it is estimated that about 1 million children in the United States live with adoptive parents and that between 2 and 4 percent of American families include an adopted child[8]—that's about 120,000 adoptions each year.[9] Lots of couples have successfully adopted children to build their family; you can too.

Some Basic Things to Think About

If you choose the option of adoption, take some time to look where you're going before you leap. There are lots of decisions to be made and matters you and your partner will have to come to agreement on before you can hope to manage the adoption process successfully. You should read several of the wonderful books that have been written about adoption, go online to gather the latest on government regulations (which vary wildly from state to state), and learn all the ins and outs of this very important life step. (See the box on page 194 for some adoption resources.) This section in this one chapter will give you a general overview, but it's only a start.

One of the first things you'll need to think carefully about is the type of adoption you're interested in. Your options fall into three basic categories: domestic, international, and an older "waiting child" from the public social services system.

Domestic Adoptions

Domestic adoptions place children from the United States (usually newborns and infants) with adoptive parents within 1 to 3 years of application. If you're interested in a domestic adoption, you'll also need to decide whether you want to adopt privately (also called independently) or use an agency. In a private adoption there is no "middleman." You will find your own birth mother and make adoption arrangements. You may use the help of your minister, your lawyer, a counselor, a doctor, or a friend—people who are not licensed by the state as an adoption agency. You may find your baby through word-of-mouth referrals, the Internet, or newspaper ads.

If you're interested in a domestic adoption, you'll also need to decide whether you want to adopt privately (also called independently) or use an agency.

On the other hand, you may sign up with an adoption agency, which can be public or private, profit or nonprofit. In any case, make sure the agency is licensed by the state. These agencies help you through each step of the adoption process and are available for domestic, international, or foster care children.

International Adoptions

One of the fastest ways to adopt an infant is through international adoptions—the adoption by an American couple of a child born outside the United States. These children are generally about 3 months to 2 years old, and the process takes about 9 to 12 months from the time of application to the time of adoption.

International adoptions have become a very popular adoption choice. The number of children adopted from other countries more than doubled in a 10-year period—from 8,102 in 1989 to 16,396 in 1999. More than half of the 1999 adoptees were from four countries: Russia, China, South Korea, and Guatemala.[10] If you choose this type of adoption, you will need to find and sign on with an adoption agency that specializes in international adoptions to help you complete the complex requirements and paperwork involved.

Waiting-Child Adoptions

Children in the public child welfare system are "waiting" to find permanent homes. Most are older, school-age children and difficult-to-place children (children who often are minorities, have physical or mental disabilities, have siblings who must be placed together, or have special medical and emotional needs). They are available through public and private welfare agencies and can usually be adopted more quickly than other children.

Eileen Murphy, who has founded a coaching company in Michigan called Family Transitions Coaching (www.familytransitions.org), adopted two older children through the public foster care system and is very aware of both the joys and difficulties involved in this decision. "Six years ago," says Eileen, "my husband, Mike, and I decided to adopt school-age children from the foster care system because the need was so great. But at first we were rejected as adoptive parents because we couldn't prove that we were infertile, which to me seemed like the most ludicrous thing on the planet! If we were able to have our own kids, we probably would not be asking for one of these children." The representatives from the state foster program told Murphy and her husband that they needed their infertility confirmed because they worried that if adoptive couples then had their own biological child, they would not want the adopted child. Despite years of unsuccessfully trying to have children, for this couple this fact was not so easy to prove.

"The doctors, as I learned very quickly," recalls Murphy, "don't want to say someone absolutely can't have children because if they say that and then somehow a woman ends up pregnant, they're concerned about being sued." So unlike most couples, Murphy and her husband began aggressive infertility testing *after* they decided to adopt. "The stress of all these tests was terrible to go through after making a decision to adopt, but that was what we had to do." Finally, one of the three doctors Murphy had seen agreed to state in writing that it would be extremely unlikely that she would be able to bear children. She and her husband were finally cleared for adoption.

The rules and regulations governing adoption through the welfare system are different state to state, so you have to investigate carefully on your own, but in any state, you'll find that adopting children from the foster care system has issues to consider that are different from domestic or international adoptions. "I'm an advocate for adopting older kids from the welfare system," says Murphy, "but only if you really know what you're getting into. The vast majority of the older children who are in the foster care system have been abused. In some ways, it's easier to adopt an older child because there's no waiting list, but you have to be committed to totally changing a child's life.

In any state, you'll find that adopting children from the foster care system has issues to consider that are different from domestic or international adoptions.

"You also have to realize that that child may never bond with you, which is the hardest part," Murphy adds. "It takes a lot of time, patience, and energy to make a family out of an older child adoption. Six years ago we adopted two older children (siblings) who were taken from their parents at ages 4 and 6; we adopted them at ages 6 and 8. One adjusted very quickly and very well, and his older sister, who was sexually abused, has had great difficulty learning how to trust again.

"Ours isn't a June and Ward Cleaver household," she continues, "and most older-child adoptions are not. I deal with a lot of families

Adoption Resource Referrals

These are useful sources of advice, support, and information:

Adoptive Families of America

3333 Highway 100 North
Minneapolis, MN 55422
Phone: (800) 372-3300
Web site: www.adoptivefam.org

This organization will refer you to a local adoptive-parents support group and send you how-to materials, including its magazine *Adoptive Families*.

The National Adoption Information Clearinghouse

5540 Nicholson Lane, Suite 300
Rockville, MD 20852
Phone: (301) 231-6512
Web site: www.casanet.org/library/adoption/naic.htm

This agency makes referrals and mails out many free fact sheets.

The American Academy of Adoption Attorneys

P.O. Box 33053
Washington, D.C. 20033
Web site: www.adoptionattorneys.com

This organization offers a directory of its members.

Helpful Web sites include these:

www.adoption.com
www.parentprofiles.com
www.adoptablekids.com
www.adoptionnetworking.com
www.adoptionsites.com

and communication issues, and over and over again I hear couples say, 'We adopted an older child because we really wanted a family right away and this seemed like the easiest way to make that happen.' We all find out quickly that it's not 'easy.' Some social workers who have been around a while will be realistic with you and try to make sure that you understand what you're getting into. Others are eternally optimistic and don't explain that there may be a downside. My husband and I both have psychology and education backgrounds, and we did a lot of studying before we made up our minds. We read a lot and talked to several people who had been through this. We knew precisely what we were doing, and I believe that this preparation is the reason our family is still together."

Become Empowered Before You Begin

Peter Gibbs, M.A., L.M.F.T., is the director of the Center for Adoption Research at the University of Massachusetts. With past experience as a clinician, an adoption consultant, and the director of an adoption agency, Gibbs sees a strong need for prospective adoptive couples to find ways to feel empowered and active in the adoption process.

"Couples who are just coming off medical infertility treatments have been through an experience that is brutal, invasive, and insensitive to any other issues in life. I've gone through this myself," Gibbs admits, "and so I know that many couples come out feeling wiped out emotionally and financially and are very vulnerable. They have just faced the greatest disappointment of their life and now need to gear up again to begin the adoption process—something most know very little about. It's very important for them to become proactively engaged in this next step toward parenthood and to establish a sense of control in the experience."

Gibbs acknowledges that there are many aspects of adoption over which the prospective parents simply have no control, and sometimes things go wrong. Some adoption plans fail, and there's nothing anyone can do to "fix" it. But he believes that the likelihood of failure can be reduced if the prospective parents are proactive when laying the groundwork right in the beginning.

"When a couple calls me as they are transitioning from infertility treatments to the adoption process, they are often very concerned about time," Gibbs says. "They want to know where they should go and what they should do right away. I understand the urgency, but at the front end of the adoption process, it is really important to do your homework first. The time spent investigating all aspects of adoption is a good investment even in the face of your feelings of urgency.

The likelihood of failure can be reduced if the prospective parents are proactive when laying the groundwork right in the beginning.

"As you go down the road of adoption," Gibbs continues, "because you're dealing with the lives of human beings, things will come up that you didn't plan on (yes, they always will!). When this happens, it will raise questions such as 'Did I make the right choice?' 'Can the program I am working with be trusted?' 'Should I have used some other approach?' If you have done the work at the beginning to be as clear as you can be about whom you are working with and what you're getting into, you will have more confidence in your informed choice. This in itself is empowering."

So before you open the yellow pages and dial up an adoption agency, do your homework. Here are six steps that Gibbs suggests you take as you begin this journey:

- Read everything you can find on the subject so you understand the stages of the process. Many good books about adoption are available, and Web sites are full of information. You can also find periodical articles in many online databases. Read!

- Go to orientation meetings offered by various adoption agencies and programs. This gives you a good chance not only to gather valuable information but also to get a feel for their style.

- Ask lots of questions. Don't worry about appearing difficult or uninformed; many others in the room share the same questions and concerns. Addressing your concerns in the beginning can avoid many problems and misunderstandings later in the process. (See the list of questions on page 199.)

- Look for advocacy and support groups that will encourage and help you and that can lead you to the resources you need.

- Clarify your own desires and needs. Do you want a newborn child? A domestic or international child? Would you be willing to explore the adoption of an older child? Do you have cultural, ethnic, or nationality preferences? What kind of relationship do you expect to have with the birth parents? That is, would you like an open adoption in which you and the birth parent(s) maintain a level of direct contact? Or would you prefer a more confidential adoption in which there is limited or perhaps indirect contact through intermediaries such as the program that made the placement? How much time, effort, and money are you willing to put into this process?

- Most important, talk to as many people as possible who have been through the adoption process. They are the real experts.

> *You must try to explore and answer your own questions before you put yourself in a position where these important issues may be decided for you.*

You must try to explore and answer your own questions before you put yourself in a position where these important issues may be decided for you. Of course, your feelings and desires don't have to be set in stone before you go to formally apply for adoption—you are on a learning journey. But you should have a good idea about how you feel about these important issues. Right in the beginning you want to build your capacity for engaging, understanding, and asking the right questions.

Once you have reviewed the facts and understand as much as possible what you're in for, then it's time to choose the adoption agency or program. "The way an adoption is handled varies dramatically from the various agencies, lawyers, and facilitators," says Gibbs. "Differences in style and approach have much to do with the kind of experiences people have. When looking for adoption resources, everyone is concerned about issues like the kind of child who is available for placement through that resource, how long the process takes, and how much it costs. But too often they overlook the fact that each agency or program has a unique personality that should match the couple's personality. They need to find the right fit in order to feel confident.

"I believe that the way a person goes through the adoption process has an impact on how they feel about themselves as parents and about their child," Gibbs adds. "If the process is perceived as a brutal, horrific experience, that is hard to separate from your feelings about how your family was formed. The couple needs to understand that they control the choice of agency or program and that choice should be made very carefully. Too often after coming away from infertility treatments where they have had so little control over what's happening, they are again ready to hand over the decisions that need to be made to anyone who says, 'I can help you.'"

Feeling empowered when choosing an agency or program can be difficult when you also want to be "approved." You don't want to annoy a representative of the adoption agency who might put you on the end of the list. You don't want the adoption lawyer to feel you're too pushy or demanding. And so you may tend to become passive and let other people tell you what's best. It is important to know that you have the right to ask anything. You don't have the right to a satisfactory answer, but you do have a right to an honest response to all your questions without worrying about being "blackballed." Any agency, program, or consultant who isn't open to talking, discussing, and exploring isn't the right one for you.

Yes, there are a lot of things that are out of your control during the adoption process, but you definitely want to identify the things that are in your control and be in a position to make the best decisions you can with the best information you can get. "That's your investment at

General Questions to Ask About Adoption

In his book, *Adopting in Massachusetts,* Peter Gibbs suggests that you ask the following questions before signing up with any adoption agency:

- How many children were placed in the last 2 years for specific programs?

- Are there any restrictions that apply to applicants?

- What is the typical total cost for adopting? What services are included in the fixed fees? What fees are variable? What has been the highest total cost? Is there a sliding-fee scale for services based on income?

- Is there a wait to begin a home study?

- What is the average time to wait for placement?

- What types of educational programs are offered for preadoptive and adoptive families?

- How does the matching process work?

- What kind of information does the agency provide regarding the health, development, and history of children and birth parents? When do they provide this?

- Can applicants talk with other families who have used the agency's services?

- What happens if you turn down a match/placement opportunity?

- What pre- and post-placement support services are available?

- What kind of prenatal and early infancy information is available?

Source: Adopting in Massachusetts, senior editor Peter Gibbs (Center for Adoption Research, University of Massachusetts, 2000). Reprinted with permission from the Center for Adoption Research.

the front end," Gibbs says. "Understand in advance, as best you can, what you can control to help reach your goal and what you cannot."

This understanding alone will make the adoption process run far smoother than if you make the mistake of calling the first agency you happen upon and hand over all the decision-making power. "Adopting is a voluntary activity," says Gibbs. "It should never make you feel like a passive victim."

Two Happy Endings

Alice has twice adopted infants through the domestic adoption process with a Catholic Charities agency in Texas. Now her boys are 18 and 15 years old, and as she looks back at the way her family was built, she is still amazed that after all her struggles and worries, things have worked out as they should.

At age 27, Alice learned she had endometriosis and was infertile. She went through several years of treatment that included medications and surgery, but she remained infertile with hormonal imbalances and soon found that her husband, Joe, had low sperm motility. It wasn't long before the doctors were talking about artificial insemination, and that's when Alice and Joe had a long, sit-down talk.

"The medications were very hard on my body," Alice remembers, "and they caused me to feel emotionally dead—no highs, no lows, and no sexual feelings. I had had enough. Besides, we really didn't want to conceive a child with ART or surrogacy, and we knew in our hearts that there were children out there who needed us just as much as we needed them, so we felt a lot more comfortable with the idea of adoption than we did with assisted reproduction. I'm not saying it was easy to give up my dream of having a natural child. I went through a difficult grieving period, and now, 18 years later, I still have times when I feel the loss. But there was never a moment in time when it occurred to me that I would remain childless."

It took Alice and Joe about 2 years from the time they were accepted by an agency to the time they brought their week-old infant into their home. They had no direct contact with the birth mother, but this was a partially open adoption in which both the birth parents and the adoptive parents could write letters to each other that were delivered through the adoption agency. (In this case, the letters from the birth mother stopped coming within the first year.)

Soon the baby grew into a happy 2-year-old who had progressed smoothly through each stage of babyhood. At this point, Alice and her husband decided to begin the process again. Within the following year, they brought home a 3-month-old infant son.

This child had been placed in foster care immediately after birth because the parental rights paperwork was incomplete. At 3 months, the adoption case workers felt it was safe to place the child, but the adoption was not legally finalized for another 3 months. Of course, those were a long and sometimes anxious 3 months, but eventually everything fell into place and the adoption was finalized.

It took Alice and Joe about 2 years from the time they were accepted by an agency to the time they brought their week-old infant into their home.

Even though everything worked out fine and Alice couldn't love her boys more if they were her natural children, there's no denying that a sense of loss still pops up at unexpected times in various ways. "I can't help but look at my nieces and nephews sometimes and notice the strong family resemblance," she admits. "In fact, my one niece has my toes! My Irish background and my husband's German features do not in any way match my children's, who both are of Hispanic heritage.

"I also struggle with the learning problems my boys have had," Alice adds. "I guess because my husband and I had always been straight-A students, I imagined our birth children as bright and eager learners.

"It took time, but I've come to the realization that no parent can predict the path a child will take, whether a natural birth child or an adopted child. I've also learned to fully enjoy the surprises that come with the unknown. My boys each came to us as a unique package, and we had no expectations about what each one 'should' be. Unlike many natural parents, we did not expect that they would inherit our own interests and talents. There was no feeling that because these boys were in our family they would naturally be great athletes, or accomplished musicians, or anything like that. I was actually looking forward to finding out if they would bring to our family talents that no one had ever had before! It's been a wonderful process watching them grow and develop into the fine young men they've become."

After all has been said and done, Alice has no doubts that adoption was the right decision for her. "I can't help but believe," she says, "that each adoption was a match directed by God. I believe that these were children who needed somebody like me and their dad to come along at just that time. They would not have grown and developed as they have if we had not been looking for a child just when they were looking for parents. I feel deeply that building a family through adoption is not second best. It has its own unique joys."

Mandy, too, is an adoptive mom who is looking forward to the surprises that will come as she watches her young son grow and develop. During her years as a publicist for an infertility center, Mandy had never imagined in her wildest dreams that someday she would suffer the heartache of failed IUI and IVF cycles and end up adopting a child from Russia. But that is what life has handed her, and now she feels quite blessed.

While handling public relations for the center, Mandy believed that assisted reproduction was absolutely wonderful, like a storybook ending for infertile couples. "But then when I actually went through it because I had polycystic ovaries and my husband, Mark, had low sperm count," she says, "I found that I no longer felt comfortable perpetuating the idea that assisted reproductive technologies are the absolute answers to infertility problems. In the majority of cases, they are not."

In Mandy's case, both artificial insemination and IVF with intracytoplasmic sperm injection failed. Cycles were canceled, she was hospitalized with hyperstimulation, her kidneys failed, and her 29 frozen embryos didn't survive the thaw when she was ready to try again. "That was it for me!" says Mandy. "No more IVFs. I went through all this knowing that I could end up with nothing in the end. And so when I began to think about adoption (which I did every time my husband was injecting me with fertility drugs), I found I really liked the idea that at least offered the promise of a child.

"On the day that I got the negative results of my last pregnancy test," Mandy continues, "that was the official end of my hope for a birth child. I went on the Web site message board that I had joined for support during my treatments, and I told everyone that I was finished and was going to adopt. I logged off and then ran around the house gathering up all the drugs and injection packets, and I threw them all away. I felt really happy. I knew that I wanted to be a mom far more than I wanted to be pregnant. From that moment on, all my energies were focused on the adoption process."

Mandy and Mark started to explore adoption options in March, and in November they were on their way to Russia to pick up their 13-month-old son. "It was a wonderful experience because we had to spend 3 weeks there. It was great quality, one-on-one time with our new son."

Today, Ilya is 3 years old, and Mandy is one of the happiest moms on Earth. "I just want to go up to people struggling through infertility treatments and tell them not to do it," she says. "Of course, everyone has to reach the point of realization on their own, but I'd love them all to see how happy they could be with an adopted child. We always wanted just one child, and now I have him. I have no desire to get pregnant and would probably resent the intrusion on our little family unit. Life is perfect for us just the way it is."

> *I knew that I wanted to be a mom far more than I wanted to be pregnant.*
>
> —MANDY

A Word of Caution

As wonderful as adoption has been for Alice and Mandy, there certainly are reasons for caution and care before choosing this option. Mary Sullivan, M.S.W., a clinical social worker teaching a class through RESOLVE of Illinois called "The ABCs of Adoption," feels it is important that couples understand the good and the bad of adoption before they make any decisions. Her involvement in this field began with her own infertility and her decision to adopt at the age of 35.

"Making the decision to end infertility treatment," recalls Mary, "is like ending life support. You're pulling the plug on the child you have created in your mind. It's like saying, 'I'm not going to keep that child alive anymore.' This is a very difficult, conscious decision that is hard to make." The first few months after making that decision were especially bleak for Mary. "I felt like I was in mourning," she remembers. "I was going through the motions of my life, but that's all." Mary understands why coming off that experience, many couples are too ready to make quick decisions about adoption before they've had time to explore all the consequences.

> *It is important that couples understand the good and the bad of adoption before they make any decisions.*

After 4 years of failed infertility treatments, Mary and her husband got a phone call from a relative who knew a pregnant teenager. She wanted to know whether Mary would be interested in adopting. "My husband's quick reaction was, 'No, we really don't want to go that route,' but I was in the background saying, 'Wait. Let's talk about this.'" That call opened up the door to the next step toward parenting for the couple, which (as they soon found out) can be fraught with pitfalls. They began the process of getting themselves licensed, but then the birth mother decided to parent her baby herself. "I now know that it's really quite common for this to happen," says Mary, "but it's still very upsetting."

After years of having hopes dashed after every attempt at assisted reproduction, infertile couples who now hope their prayers will be answered through adoption find out that this route can also have its own disappointments. But at least this experience got Mary and her husband into the adoption process.

Now it was decision time, and there was much to learn. After studying all the adoption options, in the end Mary and her husband agreed that they wanted to adopt domestically because they wanted a newborn, they wanted an open adoption, and they wanted to find their own birth mother. With the help of an adoption consultant and a lawyer, they began to advertise in newspapers and joined several adoption and education support groups to help them better understand what to expect and what to do next.

> *Infertile couples who now hope their prayers will be answered through adoption find out that this route can also have its own disappointments.*

Mary's son's birth mother answered one of the newspaper ads. "We exchanged information," she remembers. "Then we didn't hear any more from her. Several weeks later we were told that there was a different birth mother who had read our file and wanted to place her baby with us. The baby was already born, and we were really excited about becoming parents immediately. But by the next morning, the second birth mother had changed her mind, and that deal was off. A few hours later our consultant called back and said they had just heard from the first birth mother who had contacted us. She was ready to commit to adoption. I felt so confused. It was just impossible for me to believe that I would ever become a mother."

But this time it did happen. Mary and her husband arrived at the hospital 5 minutes after their son was born. Two days later after the birth parents had surrendered their parental rights, the baby was placed with Mary and her husband.

Four years after this first adoption, the couple decided to adopt a second child. Taking another deep breath, they headed back into the adoption process. They were soon contacted by someone who knew a pregnant woman who was looking for adoptive parents. After talking with that birth mother on the phone, they agreed to meet, and Mary and her husband flew to the state where she lived. They spent a day with her and the birth father, after which the birth mother agreed to place the baby with them. But it wasn't long before she had a change of heart, and Mary was again left angry and confused.

When the next call came, Mary wasn't sure that she wanted to try this again, but she agreed to go through the motions to see what would happen. This baby was born a month early at 4 pounds, 5 ounces, and the two teen parents suddenly thought they might keep her. Again, the anxious waiting began.

At the last moment, this tiny baby girl was handed over to Mary and her husband. Because of her prematurity and size, this baby had a lot of needs. She needed time to grow and many medical professionals to monitor her progress. "In fact," admits Mary, "although we adore our children and think they are both wonderful in so many ways, both of them have a lot of special needs, and I can't say that I am nearly the cheerleader for adoption that I once was. Adopting may be the only way some people can become parents, but it is very different from having a biological child in very significant ways. I think it's really important for people to appreciate that before they make any final decisions.

"Whether you ever have contact with the birth parents or not or whether you adopt from this country or another, this child has other parents who contributed the genetic material that makes up the child," she adds. "Life does not prepare us to understand and accept this. It's a huge leap to agree to parent a child that someone else gave birth to. There are major ramifications to consider when you can't truly know the full medical or prenatal background that went into making this child.

"In my experience, both personally and professionally, the fact is you can't begin to predict what will reveal itself over time. Although no parents can order up a perfectly healthy child, in the realm of adoption, you are more at risk for certain things like babies who are born with the effects of prenatal exposure to drugs and alcohol. It's important to know this ahead of time and be ready for that possibility. Too many adoption agencies are not up-front about this and I think that's irresponsible. The fact is that fetal alcohol exposure is high

Adoption Advice

"It's very normal to have trouble navigating the adoption process. In addition to becoming well educated about the mechanics of adoption, some people also find it useful to get counseling from an independent professional therapist who is knowledgeable about adoption. We found therapy very helpful."

Mary Sullivan, M.S.W., a clinical social worker

among many women who place their babies for adoption, and this affects the mental and physical health of the child. It's also a fact that birth mothers have a right to change their mind and parent their babies themselves. Prospective parents need to know and accept this to make an informed decision."

It's true, as Mary Sullivan learned, that you can't totally prevent bad things from happening in an adoption. But all experts involved in the adoption process agree that by being educated and proactive you can contribute to the best possible outcome.

NONPARENTING

Some infertile couples, for various personal reasons, do not want to create a family using donor eggs or sperm, surrogacy, or adoption. Instead, they choose the option of nonparenting. This choice can be a particularly difficult one. While some couples can easily adapt to this lifestyle, others struggle for years with the pain of this loss.

Serafina Corsello, M.D., founder of the Corsello Centers for Complementary-Alternative Medicine in New York City, is a psychiatrist who has worked with many infertile women. Her integrative mind-body program has helped many achieve their dream of conception, but she also counsels those who make the decision to forego the dream of parenting and move on to a life without children. "Many of these women," Dr. Corsello says, "experience the stages of grief common to those suffering a loss through death." These stages, explored by Elisabeth Kübler-Ross in her book, *On Death and Dying*, include the following:

1. **Denial and isolation.** In this stage, you may intellectually know nonparenting is best for you, but you haven't accepted that fact emotionally yet and may have trouble dealing with the reality of the outer world.

2. **Anger.** You may feel anger, not only at being infertile but at everyone and everything around you. Nothing seems fair, right, or worthwhile. If the anger is internalized over a long period, you may find yourself slipping into the next stage: depression.

3. **Depression.** Being clinically depressed is different from being sad. Although normal sadness can cause changes in appetite, sleeping habits, and other behaviors, depression may show itself in extremes of behavior: not eating or eating too much, not sleeping or sleeping too much, withdrawing completely or talking incessantly, or being extremely hostile or totally apathetic. If these extremes continue for a prolonged time (more than 2 weeks), clinical depression may be the culprit, and professional help is advised.

4. **Acceptance.** At this stage, you can move forward to build a life for yourself and your partner that does not include the child of your dreams.

(Note: Bargaining is also a common stage in the grief process, but by the time infertile couples choose nonparenting, they have already played all their bargaining chips: "I will give up smoking and drinking if it will make me fertile." "I will put my body through any kind of medical procedure if it will improve my fertility." And so on.)

Almost all of us pass through these stages during times of great loss, though not necessarily in any specific order, and sometimes we go through more than one stage simultaneously or jump back and forth from one to another. "The goal," says Dr. Corsello, "is to reach the level of acceptance where the couple is content to live with the love and support of each other and look forward to what the future holds for the two of them. But this is not always easy to do. After years of spending money and time, and doing injections, and taking tests, and submitting to fertility treatments, and putting the body through hell, now how do you stop and say, 'I'm ready to give up this plan for my life and look for another one equally as valuable'?"

The key to finding a new life direction, according to Dr. Corsello, is in something called *social reengineering*. "In the past," she says, "you may have been organizing your life around your dream family that included a baby. You may have been going through certain medical procedures; you may have been saving money for the child's upbringing or college education; you may have been changing your career goals to accommodate the baby. Now, all that changes. You need to engineer a new reality and create a positive outlook."

To begin shaping this new reality, Dr. Corsello recommends a mental exercise that can help you implant pleasant images to accompany your new lifestyle. "Make a list," she says, "of all the things you would be doing if you had had children, raised them to adulthood, and were now living on your own with your partner. How would you be spending your life? Would you travel? Would you go to the opera? Would you buy season tickets to see a sports team? Would you volunteer your time to help others? These are the things that you can do right now to begin to feel fulfilled and productive."

Building relationships with other nonparenting couples is another positive step you can take toward creating your new life. People who

> *The key to finding a new life direction, according to Dr. Serafina Corsello, is in something called* social reengineering.

are childfree (whether by choice or chance) have different interests, hobbies, and pastimes than those involved in the time-intensive job of parenting. Seek out people at work, in your community or church, or through clubs and organizations who enjoy their lives without children—there are a lot of people like this in the world around you. For a variety of reasons, such as effective birth control, later marriages, career opportunities, and rising infertility rates, the number of women without children has increased dramatically over the past 30 years—and the trend continues. According to an article in *American Demographics*, the number of childless couples will increase by 4 percent by 2010.[11]

In other words, you are not alone. You can begin chatting today with other people in the same circumstance (real adults who can talk about things other than babies and children!) on these two online sites: (1) Childless by Choice at www.Now2000.com/cbc and (2) No Kidding! at www.nokidding.net.

As you begin to reengineer your life, be kind to yourself and don't expect miracles. Even infertile childless couples who have lived long and fulfilled lives admit that they feel a lingering sense of loss even years later. Like the death of a loved one, the sense of sadness and grief that accompanies the death of the dream of parenting is something that will never disappear completely. But it does ease over time when you find new ways to compensate for this loss.

> *Once a state of acceptance is reached, you can then move forward to the empowering realization that life can still be wonderful and fulfilling.*

However, if you simply can't envision a worthwhile and pleasant life for yourself without your own children, it would be wise to seek the help of a professional counselor. Dr. Corsello agrees and says, "For some people, doing the work of social reengineering by themselves is like being in a deep hole and hearing other people say, 'Cheer up and get yourself out of that hole.' You need somebody to throw you a rope and help you climb out." Many counselors and therapists are specially trained in helping infertile couples accept a life without children. Once this state of acceptance is reached, you can then move forward to the empowering realization that life can still be wonderful and fulfilling.

This is the place where Shelia and Paul have finally landed. After 7 years of battling infertility and almost destroying their marriage, this couple decided it was time to stop and look in a new direction for life goals. "I'm not saying this was an easy choice," admits Shelia. "I did a lot of crying when we told our doctor that we would not be trying any more infertility treatments. We had spent a fortune and walked away empty-handed, and I thought there was nothing in life to look forward to anymore.

"I don't know exactly what made me see things in a more positive way, but I do remember one morning looking at my husband as we were getting ready to leave for work and thinking, 'I am so lucky. I have this good man as a husband. We both have our health and a whole lifetime of possibilities in front of us. How awful it will be if we look back in our old age and see years spent grieving for the life we couldn't have.' I think it was that fear of ruining the possibility of a good life that made me reevaluate the time and energy I had been putting into being angry and sad."

Resource Referral

You can contact the following organization to find a therapist who specializes in helping infertile couples:

National Mental Health Association
1021 Prince Street
Alexandria, VA 22314
Phone: (800) 969-6642
Web site: www.nmha.org

Life has changed for Shelia and Paul since that day she decided that she had spent enough time grieving for what couldn't be. "I've actually found that I really enjoy doing things with and for my sister's children and my own godchild. Instead of avoiding them because they remind me of my own failing, now I feel I've become important to them, and I know I give them so many things that their own parents simply can't—like undivided attention, free-for-all spoiling rights, and an objective view in problem situations. I love them all dearly, and they enrich my life—a life that I can now see has great value spent with the man I love doing the things that bring us happiness and contentment."

KEEPING IT TOGETHER

No matter how you decide to build your future family, you will need to keep yourself mentally and emotionally strong in very difficult circumstances. The next chapter will give you some insights into the relationship between mental health and fertility, with some easy exercises that can help you keep yourself together.

CHAPTER 6

The Mind, the Body, and Infertility

INFERTILITY THROWS MUCH attention on your physical body. Blood tests, semen samples, medical procedures, fertility drugs, and a variety of assisted reproductive technologies take up your time, energy, and focus. Unfortunately, in the process, something vital to life is often compromised: your emotional and mental health.

You don't need to be told that being infertile is tough on your psyche. This is something that some say feels like a death—the death of dreams and plans. It is the loss of control over your life's direction and destiny. It brings with it negative feelings such as anger, rage, guilt, and envy that easily get out of control. Not surprisingly, marital, family, and social relationships can also suffer.

This definitely is not the life you had planned for yourself, yet it's the only one you've got. Now your ability to accept it, deal with it, and move forward will ultimately influence the quality of that life. This chapter will take a look at the mind–body connection in infertility and offer you some tips for managing its mental and emotional aspects. In some cases, this kind of control can improve your state of fertility, but most important, in all cases, it will improve the quality of the life you live.

EMOTIONALLY BATTERED

When 32-year-old Ann finishes her graduate studies in clinical psychology, she would like to counsel women dealing with the very difficult emotions tied to infertility. She knows firsthand just how they feel. When she married her 34-year-old husband, David, they expected to hold their first child in their arms within the next year. Now 3 years later, they've been through, up, down, and around the emotional struggle of trying to have that baby. Ann spent 1 year taking her temperature, tracking her cervical mucus, changing sex positions, and eating the foods she was told would make an egg stick to her uterus. She and David gave up alcohol and cut down on caffeine, and David took up drinking orange juice and even changed his style of underwear. "Many of the things we've done," laughs Ann, "border on the superstitious, but we needed to feel that we had some sense of control." After 6 months, Ann became pregnant—but it was an ectopic pregnancy. "The emotional pain of having this failed pregnancy was absolutely traumatic. I didn't want to have anything more to do with doctors and testing, so we went through one more year of trying to conceive naturally but with no success."

Even though nothing good was happening, Ann was convinced that everything was okay. "I was frustrated that it was taking so long when other people could just look at each other and get pregnant," she admits. "But I had never let myself even consider that I could have some real problem." Then Ann finally went for medical testing and learned that she had blocked fallopian tubes. "I was devastated," she remembers. "It was just crushing. I'm a high achiever, and I'm used to passing tests very easily. I couldn't believe I failed this one."

The first few weeks were just awful for Ann, and made more so by the fact that a good friend and her 10-month-old daughter were staying at Ann's home for a couple of weeks when she got the news. Seeing this baby every day intensified the pain. "I felt a great emptiness and a sense of mourning over the loss of my ability to have children naturally. Something very important had been taken away from me, and this little girl was a daily reminder that I could not have the one thing I wanted the most. I was completely depressed for about a month."

Only those who have been diagnosed as infertile know how devastating this pronouncement can be. And only these couples know how they each, in their individual way, pull out of it and move on. For Ann, her grief was eventually replaced by practical questions. What do we do now? What exactly is IVF? Can we afford it? Who do we go to? "We got into an action mode of trying to do something, and this gave us back some control over the situation," says Ann. "I began to do some reading; I got answers from my insurance company; I began to make calls to different doctors for information. Finding out that it wasn't completely hopeless because technology could help us have our own child put me back on my feet." But unfortunately, not for long.

> *Only those who have been diagnosed as infertile know how devastating this pronouncement can be. And only these couples know how they each, in their individual way, pull out of it and move on.*

"We have finished three IVF cycles and almost had our baby," says Ann sadly. "I did get pregnant after the third one but then miscarried after 8 weeks. I've been really battered by this. I feel like I've been beaten left and right. The pain of this loss was almost unbearable for me even though I had tried to be so emotionally cautious. After getting the positive pregnancy result, I was exhilarated for about an hour—then the anxiety kicked in. I knew I could lose this baby, and so I settled for cautious happiness. But still, losing the baby was heartbreaking. We had worked so hard for 3 years to get to that point, and now we were back where we started."

David has been very supportive, but Ann sees that his emotional reactions are different than hers. "My husband is very involved in this process," she says. "He comes to every doctor's appointment; he's with me for every blood test, every ultrasound, every retrieval and transfer. But I think that because I am so emotionally charged, he tries to keep himself separated from the strong feelings so he can better take care of me. But I worry about him. I tend to look for support from others, but he keeps things bottled up, and I have this feeling that one day this may have an effect on him."

Ann still struggles most with the issue of fairness. "I just don't understand why this has happened to me. No one can give me a reason why my tubes are blocked. There is no logical reason in the world why my tubes are blocked. I can't find any larger meaning for this in my life. I can't help asking, 'Why me?' This situation brings out the worst in me and it intensifies and highlights so many awful feelings—especially my darkest, blackest feelings of envy. Envy is an ugly feeling at any time, but it's so hard to see my friends moving on to having their second child. Sometimes I'm convinced that no one can understand what I'm going through or know what this feels like. It's just awful."

Ann and David continue to hope for a baby of their own. In the meantime, they have adopted two loving cats. "They've helped us cope with not having a little one around," Ann says sadly with a shrug.

Men's Self-Esteem

A study reported in the *British Medical Journal* found that subfertile men had lower self-esteem and were more anxious than a control group with no known fertility problems. In a study of men attending a specialist male subfertility clinic, researchers found them experiencing high levels of anxiety, feeling "less of a man," and blaming themselves for the subfertility. Life satisfaction was less than they perceived it would be if they had a baby.[1]

THE IMPACT ON PERSONAL RELATIONSHIPS

The impact of infertility on your relationships can be profound. When emotions are high, one wrong word or insensitive piece of advice from anyone—spouse, parent, or friend—can send you tumbling down into a spiral of anger, resentment, and even hate. This response usually happens, unfortunately, at just the time when you need the support and encouragement of loved ones the most. Because keeping your relationships in good shape will help keep your mind at ease, it's important to try to understand the other's point of view, communicate your own needs, and work together to get through this life experience.

Family and Friends

How much information about your infertility you give to your family and friends depends on the kind of relationship you have with each person. If your parents, siblings, and close friends have in the past been supportive when you faced a difficult situation, you may want to let them know what you're going through so you have someone else besides your partner to talk to and to gain objective viewpoints from. On the other hand, if your family and friends tend to pry or be insensitive, or if you feel a sense of shame or guilt about your infertility, you may not want to let anyone know what's going on.

> *Because keeping your relationships in good shape will help keep your mind at ease, it's important to try to understand the other's point of view, communicate your own needs, and work together to get through this life experience.*

What's most important, according to Erin Kramer, president of RESOLVE of the Washington, D.C., metropolitan area, is that you and your spouse talk about who you will and will not discuss your infertility with. "If the couple hasn't talked about this in advance," she cautions, "one member of the couple might be going out telling everyone before finding out that the spouse did not want to share that information with anyone. Get together with your partner and decide exactly who you both feel comfortable sharing this news with and how much you will tell."

Some of the pressure you might feel to tell family and friends about the state of your fertility comes from the insensitive question, "So, when are you two going to have a baby?" To handle this intrusive comment with style and aplomb, you'll need to think in advance about what you want to say. If the question is asked by a nosey relative with whom you do not want to share personal details, you might say something like, "We have nothing planned for the near future, but if plans should change, we'll be sure to let you know."

If the question is asked by a close friend or family member to whom you've wanted to talk about your infertility, this question gives

> *What's most important is that you and your spouse talk about who you will and will not discuss your infertility with.*

you a good opportunity to broach the subject. You might say, "We've been trying, but we're having some difficulty." From there you can reveal as much or as little information about your situation as you'd like.

Dealing with your infertility can be particularly difficult when friends and family members are having babies all around you. Thirty-three-year-old Melinda speaks for many infertile women when she observes, "I have this theory that pregnant women follow me around. No matter where I go every day, there they are. Today I'm going to visit a friend who has just had a baby, and it's going to be hard. We haven't been as close lately as we had been because it's just so hard to listen to her good news. She got pregnant after trying for 4 months, and although I don't wish her anything but the best, it's so hard to share in her happiness.

"If I ever write a book," Melinda adds, "I'll write one that tells people how to act and what to say when you're with an infertile person. People either don't say anything or say everything that's wrong. One single friend tried to comfort me by reminding me that at least I had a husband. Another told me that if I didn't come to her baby shower, we couldn't be friends anymore. It's so hard to explain to people how you feel that you tend to withdraw and give up trying. I don't want to go to baby birthday parities. I don't want to go to the park where there are lots of kids. I don't want to talk about why I don't have children. I don't know if my family and friends can understand that."

Kramer agrees that these situations can be very difficult for infertile couples. "You have to know what situations will trigger strong emotions in you and feel comfortable about staying away from them. You may choose to make excuses or share the truth, but either way, you have a right to remove yourself from places that upset you. When I was going through my own infertility experience, baby showers were just too painful for me so I didn't go. I would either buy a gift and send it along with someone else. Or, if I weren't up to even picking out a baby gift, I would ask someone else to buy it for me or order a gift certificate online. I wanted to be happy for the pregnant friend, but it was just so painful for me because I wanted desperately to be in the same situation."

Kramer has seen many instances where the pain of infertility has disrupted close relationships. "I remember when a friend of mine was pregnant with her first child," she recalls. "She couldn't understand why her sister (who was having difficulty conceiving) couldn't be happy for her. She constantly complained that her sister wouldn't go shopping with her to buy baby items and wouldn't even talk about the baby on the phone. I tried to explain that she couldn't imagine how badly her sister wanted to be there for her but how painful it would be to do that. It's not that the sister wasn't happy about the baby, but she just couldn't face that happiness without deeply feeling her own loss. My friend had a hard time understanding this. Regardless of how other people react to your decisions, you have to know what you can and can't do and give yourself permission to avoid emotional pain."

> *You have to know what situations will trigger strong emotions in you and feel comfortable about staying away from them.*
>
> —ERIN KRAMER

Your Spouse

Infertility can throw any marriage into a spin. It is such an intimate problem that affects identity, sexuality, and self-esteem—all so closely tied to the marriage experience. But on the bright side, if the two of you can get through the rigors of infertility, you can get through anything.

> *If the two of you can get through the rigors of infertility, you can get through anything.*

In the most difficult cases, some compare infertility to the devastation felt after the death of a child. Unfortunately, it is well known that the divorce rate after the death of a child is very high; infertile couples face the same risk. Writing in *Men's Health*, Peter Landesman says bluntly, "The marriages in question either unravel or they soar. Parents-in-waiting tap previously unknown wells of emotion and compassion, or flail in pools of self-deprivation and faithlessness. There is little middle ground." Often, according to Landesman, the failure is the male's. Speaking on behalf of men, he says, "We hold ourselves responsible for the failings of our bodies. Steeped in disappointment and self-disgust, we unleash our repression on our wives. A man's weapons of choice are silence and denial."[2]

In 1983, Tracy MacNab, Ph.D., clinical director of the Marino Foundation for Integrative Medicine in Cambridge, Massachusetts, conducted a study examining infertile men's emotional responses to their infertility. Fifteen hundred questionnaires were distributed; not one was returned. It took Dr. MacNab a full year to find 30 men willing to talk about their experiences.

According to Landesman, "There is a name for this silence; it is a psychological condition: alexithymia. Its Greek derivation means 'no words for feelings.' . . . Call it what you want—denial, stoicism, alexithymia—the outcome is the same: the deprivation of honest air, silence, rejection of the self. All are poison for marriages, all obliterate self-worth."[3]

Although the road can be a treacherous one with many emotional potholes, all is not hopeless. Those couples with strong coping skills and a solid base to their marriage often come out the other end even stronger and more firmly committed. For this reason, it's important to take time to understand the experience from your spouse's point of view and learn how to communicate better so you can both find your way safely to the other side—whether that place is with a child or without.

Male Versus Female Reactions

It's inevitable that you and your partner will respond to different aspects of infertility differently. Expect it. In her book, *The Infertility Survival Guide*, Judith Daniluk, Ph.D., says, "Women frequently react with more overt emotion to their inability to produce a child. Infertile women usually experience more anxiety and depression than their infertile partners." On the other hand, Dr. Daniluk says that men, although distressed about being unable to produce a child, are more likely to be upset by their partner's obvious emotional distress and by their inability to fix the situation.[4] Men may cope by keeping themselves busy with other things and by avoiding talking about infertility.

These differences might make the woman start to believe that her husband doesn't care as much as she does about having a baby. A man might think that his wife cares more about having a baby than she does about him. Both make assumptions that hurt their relationship.

> *Men are more likely to be upset by their partner's obvious emotional distress and by their inability to fix the situation.*

Beware of Assumptions

Getting assumptions out in the open is a good way to limit the negative emotions that can strain your marriage. From now on, try to catch yourself before you state an assumption. (They often begin with the phrase "I know. . . .") Watch out for statements such as "I know you don't care about this as much as I do"; "I know you wish I would give this up"; "I know you think this is all my fault." Change it to a statement that expresses your feelings followed by a question that asks about his or her feelings. You might say, "Being a parent is important

---

A Pleasant Surprise

"You may not think your husband is really paying attention to what's going on, but he probably is. I remember when I went for a second opinion, my husband sat there and told the doctor all the things we had tried and when we did it and what the results were without missing a beat. I looked at him in total surprise. I had no idea he had been keeping track because we very rarely talk about it. It's just not something that's dinner conversation for us."

34-year-old Angela

---

to me. How do you feel?" Or, "I feel guilty about not being able to give you a child. Do you blame me for what we're going through?" Rather than carry around painful emotions like anger, guilt, and resentment based on assumptions, put them out on the table to get at the truth.

Communicate!

To keep assumptions from sabotaging your marriage, commit yourself to honest and open communication about your feelings. Your partner won't assume you hate him for not being able to give you a child if you say up-front and repeatedly afterward, "I want you to know that I love you whether or not we ever have a baby." There, now you both know. Ambivalence about having children is another common feeling. Don't feel guilty about it; discuss it with each other. These are the kind of feelings that you have to share so you're both on the same track during this journey.

While communication is important, don't overdo it. Even though it may not always seem like it, there is more to your relationship than doctor's appointments, procedures, next-step options, and so on. If you find that infertility has taken over all your daily conversations, it's time to back off and put a limit on how long you both can poke at this subject each day. Agree to a specific time—maybe 20 minutes tops— and then move on to another subject. Don't let infertility become your only point of common interest. You'll be surprised how this small change can improve your relationship.

If you find that infertility has taken over all your daily conversations, it's time to back off and put a limit on how long you both can poke at this subject each day.

REACH OUT FOR SUPPORT

Support groups can be an invaluable source of encouragement, information, and, of course, support that provides a better foundation on which to build all your other relationships. According to Lisa Rivo Peterson, Ph.D., the support group coordinator for RESOLVE of Los Angeles:

> Perhaps one of the most important benefits of participating in a support group is a decreased sense of isolation so many people feel when they are experiencing infertility. In a support group environment, feelings of anger, depression, guilt, and anxiety can be expressed, validated by others, and accepted as a normal response to the infertility crisis. Having the freedom to express negative feelings and to identify with one another helps participants to realize that they are not alone in their struggle with infertility. They can experience a sense of emotional relief from the support of others. Members who may already have a highly supportive network of family and friends can find that a group provides a place to continue to share feelings without overburdening loved ones.[5]

Knowing that you are not alone with your struggles can make life so much more bearable. Former surgeon general C. Everett Koop has noted, "My years as a medical practitioner, as well as my own first-hand experience, has taught me how important self-help groups are in assisting their members in dealing with problems, stress, hardship, and pain. . . . Today, the benefits of mutual aid are experienced by millions of people who turn to others with a similar problem to attempt to deal with their isolation, powerlessness, alienation, and the awful feeling that nobody understands."[6]

Many groups also offer more than support. Several are good places for gathering information. Members often discuss conventional and alternative treatments, for example, and trade experiences about what works and what doesn't. Some focus on learning new coping skills, such as relaxation exercises and cognitive restructuring. And almost all leave time for exchanging tips on diet, travel, family, work, and the like.

Finding a Support Group

There are many infertility support groups out there, so get the facts before you join. Some are composed of a small group of women who meet occasionally to share a cup of coffee in someone's home; others are large, structured, and highly organized. It's a good idea to investigate a few (if available in your area) and pick one that you feel most comfortable with.

You can start your search by asking your doctor whether he or she knows of any local support group. You can also call staff at a nearby city hospital and ask whether they know of or even sponsor such a group. Or, contact your local RESOLVE chapter (see the appendix for contact information).

> You can start your search by asking your doctor whether he or she knows of any local support group.

You can also use the Internet to help you find the right group. Edward Madara is the director of American Self-Help Clearinghouse—a problem-solving information bank listing over 1,000 national and international organizations across the country. His Web site (www.selfhelpgroups.org) offers information that will help you locate an infertility support group or start a group of your own.

Whether you're interested in finding an established group, forming a new group, or looking for an in-person or an online group, Madara believes that essentially four characteristics of what he calls "mutual help" groups make them what they are:

Mutual help. This is the primary dynamic process that takes place within the group—it's people helping one another and helping themselves in the process. Experiences are shared, knowledge is pooled, options are multiplied, hopes are reinforced, and efforts are joined as members strive to help one another.

Member run. When members "own" a group, they provide a sense of belonging and reflect members' felt needs. If professionals are involved (and in many cases they are), they serve in ancillary supportive roles—they are "on tap, not on top," as some groups describe it.

> **Resource Referral**
> You can contact the American Self-Help Clearinghouse by calling (973) 326-6789 or, in New Jersey, (800) FOR-MASH (for mutual aid self-help).

Composed of peers. Members share the same problem/experience, providing a powerful "you are not alone" sense of understanding, which can often lead to an almost instant sense of community at the first meeting.

Voluntary nonprofit organization. There should be no fees, and dues, if any, are minimal.

"Within a group," adds Madara, "people pool their experiences, and members of the group see positive options that they may not have thought of before."

THE STRESS–INFERTILITY CONNECTION

It's not bad enough that you're struggling physically to have a child; in addition, research strongly supports what you probably already know: The mental stress of infertility has the power to make you feel even more miserable. Here's why.

The roots of the body's physical response to stress go back to humans' primitive days. In the era of cave people, the difference between bringing an animal home to eat and being eaten by the animal was a person's ability to react quickly to danger. The human body had to be able to prepare for fight or flight at a moment's notice. To do this, the sympathetic portion of the body's autonomic nervous system released norepinephrine neurons, which influence all major organs and cause the release of adrenaline (epinephrine) from the adrenal glands. Adrenaline causes rapid heart rate, dry mouth, increased blood pressure, dilated pupils, sweating, redirection of blood flow to the muscles and away from the digestive tract and skin (causing the pale look of terror), and muscle tremor.

The problem is that this stress response, which was designed to promote the physical activity of running away or fighting, is no longer appropriate for us today. When a woman undergoing infertility treatment once again gets her monthly period, she does not need extra oxygen directed to her deep muscles, yet it happens. Even with no foe in sight and nowhere to run, our heart beats rapidly, our blood pressure rises, and our muscles tighten.

To add to this bodily assault, the stress response can cause changes in the release of hormones, so vital to fertility. This reaction happens because the fight-or-flight response originates in the hypothalamus. The hypothalamus coordinates the functions of the nervous and hormonal systems for the entire body. It is connected to the nearby pituitary gland through a short stalk of nerve fibers and controls the hormonal secretions from this gland. Research has shown that stress can indeed upset the important, delicate hormonal balance in both men and women. Such imbalances can lead to irregular or missing menstrual cycles and may cause the fallopian tubes and uterus to contract and inhibit the movement of the egg into the uterus. Stress and depression also have been implicated in the complete cessation of ovulation. Furthermore, the production of excess adrenaline in one study was linked to menstrual cycle irregularities. In men, emotional stress may be associated with abnormal sperm development.[7]

> *The reality is that, despite the known links between stress and hormone production, the medical community doesn't really know a lot about the direct relationship between stress and fertility.*

The Effects of Stress

Research has shown that women undergoing treatment for infertility have a similar, and often higher, level of stress as women dealing with life-threatening illness such as cancer and heart disease.[8] In fact, according to Rahul Sachdev, M.D., a specialist in reproductive endocrinology and infertility at the Robert Wood Johnson Medical School in New Jersey, "One study has shown that the stress levels of an infertile woman are actually similar to those of someone just told they have HIV."[9]

The reality is that, despite these known links between stress and hormone production, the medical community doesn't really know a lot about the direct relationship between stress and fertility. The studies are ongoing. But we do know that stress and other negative emotions do disrupt the quality of life. That's why relaxation exercises are highly recommended for infertile couples. There is no guarantee that they will directly result in conception and full-term pregnancy, but the possibility exists. More important, keep in mind that such exercises are an ideal way to keep yourself sane and healthy during this difficult time.

RELAX!

It's understandable that you're feeling stressed. You live on the emotional high hopes and low letdowns of each monthly menstrual cycle. But it is not absolutely necessary to let this stress take charge of your life. Wherever you may be in the process of dealing with your infertility, relaxation exercises can help you take back control of your emotional health and keep your body functioning at its peak physical level. Here are a few relaxation techniques to get you started.

Breathe Deeply

People under stress tend to breathe with their chest muscles. If you take a deep breath right now, you may find that your chest puffs out as you fill your lungs with air—this breathing habit is adding to your stress. Watch a child as he sleeps and you'll see the stomach muscles rise up with each breath as the diaphragm—not the chest—fills with air. Many adults have lost this natural breathing mechanism that is most efficient in bringing restorative oxygen to all tissues of the body.

Every day, practice breathing from your diaphragm:

1. Place one hand on your chest and one on your upper stomach.
2. As you take a deep breath in, feel the hand on your stomach rise. The hand on your chest should not rise up.
3. Let the air go. Don't push it out—let it go gently. Feel the hand on your stomach go down.

When you have the knack of diaphragm breathing, focus on the pace of your breathing. Short, shallow breaths are stressful to the body. As you practice this deep-breathing technique, change your pace to six breaths per minute. (If you check your "natural" breathing pattern right now, you may find that you're taking about 10 breaths per minute.) Take in a slow, easy breath to the count of four. Then release the breath to the count of four. Hold your breath for 2 seconds. This 10-second cycle will give you six breaths per minute.

> *Deep breathing is a strategy you can use anywhere.*

Deep breathing is a strategy you can use anywhere. No one around needs to know you're practicing a stress reduction technique. It's a technique you can engage in whenever you feel your stress level rising. Automatically, deep breathing will change your body's stress reaction.

In the beginning, you'll find that although the deep-breathing exercise is easy, your chest-breathing habit will return as soon as you're not paying attention. Give yourself a couple of weeks of practicing deep breathing just a few minutes here and there throughout the day, and soon you'll find that your body will relearn how to breathe correctly on its own.

Imagine This

To feel stress, your brain has to perceive it. The technique of mental imagery literally takes your mind off the stressful situation and focuses it on something positive, causing the brain to release brain chemicals that elevate mood and diminish stress—really!

The goal with mental imagery for relaxation is to ease the muscle tension of stress by tricking the body into thinking you're relaxed and having a good time. Sit back, close your eyes, and imagine a very pleasant incident or place. For example, some people find this kind of image soothing:

> I am stretched out on the ocean beach. The sun is warm on my body. When it gets too strong, I have an umbrella for protection. I feel the warmth of the sand on my fingertips. I see the calm ocean touching the shore. I can smell the salt of the ocean and I can taste the sea air. On my beach there's just the right number of people—I'm not crowded or lonely. On my beach there are no sand crabs or flies. I feel just wonderful. It's an ideal place that I can visit with all my senses anytime I want. Even when I'm in the middle of a crowd with my eyes wide open, I can go to my beach.

This safe place happens to be a beach—yours can be anywhere. It can be in your family room by the fireplace, the woods by a stream, the park down the street. It can be anywhere, but keep these points in mind:

- Make the place real. When you're stressed or in pain, you won't be able to relate to an alien planet.
- Involve all of your senses. Make sure all the things you touch, taste, hear, smell, and see in this environment are pleasing to you.
- Go to this place often. The more you practice increasing the quality of your image, the more you can rely on it when you're in emotional pain. It will become a practiced response.

Relax Those Muscles

In stressful situations, many people describe the way they feel as being "tied up in knots." Because of the way our muscles react to stress, this sense actually is true. Progressive muscle relaxation will help you untie the knots by teaching you how to recognize muscle tension and then how to relax the involved muscles. By practicing progressive muscle relaxation, you will learn what it feels like when stress begins to manifest itself in muscle tension. Then when your muscles do begin to tense involuntarily, you will be able to identify the problem area and stop the stress attack.

> *Progressive muscle relaxation will help you untie the knots by teaching you how to recognize muscle tension and then how to relax the involved muscles.*

To begin, tense and relax a muscle group— let's start with your right hand and arm. Press your forearm down against a table. Feel where the tension goes out through your fingertips, up into your shoulder, right into your neck. Maintain that tension for 5 to 10 seconds so you have time to feel how whole parts of your body are involved in tension. Then relax. Feel the experience of letting go—of consciously relaxing your muscles. Then move on to other muscle groups: tighten the muscles in each leg and foot, the abdomen and chest, the face, jaw, and forehead. By repeating this exercise, muscle group by muscle group throughout the body, you develop more and more control over the muscles and become increasingly sensitive and attuned to how a tense muscle and a relaxed muscle feel. Frequent repetition of short practice times throughout the day is a good way to learn this skill.

Try Biofeedback

People are quick to say, "Oh, just relax!" But the truth is that it is a rare person who can truly tell when his or her body is tense. That's why you may find biofeedback very helpful.

The Association of Applied Psychophysiology and Biofeedback (AAPB) tells us:

The word "biofeedback" was coined in late 1969 to describe laboratory procedures (developed in the 1940s) that trained research subjects to alter brain activity, blood pressure, muscle tension, heart rate, and other bodily functions that are not normally controlled voluntarily. Biofeedback is a training technique in which people are taught to improve their health and performance by using signals from their own bodies.

One common biofeedback device, for example, picks up electrical signals from the muscles. Every time muscles become tense, this device triggers a flashing light or activates a beeper. If you want to slow down the flashing or beeping, you must learn how to relax the tense muscles. After you learn to control muscle tension, you can shake off the effects of stress anywhere, anytime without being attached to the sensors.

> **Referral Resource**
>
> To find a biofeedback practitioner near you, call the AAPB in Wheat Ridge, Colorado, at (303) 422-8436, or contact the group through its Web site at www.aapb.org.

Other biological functions that are commonly measured and used in a similar way to help people learn to control their physical functioning are skin temperature, heart rate, sweat gland activity, and brainwave activity. Studies have shown that we have more control over so-called involuntary bodily functions than we once thought possible.[10]

What this means is that biofeedback helps you "see" your muscle tension and how relaxation exercises can reduce the tension that contributes to your pain.

Use Scents to Destress

Aromatherapy is a healing treatment that utilizes the essential oils of both cultivated and wild plants that emit an aroma as they evaporate. Essential oils are found in the petals (lavender), leaves (basil), wood (cedar wood), fruit (orange), seeds (sesame), roots (ginger), gum (myrrh), and resin (pine). In many cases, the oils are located in more than one part of the plant. An orange, for example, has essential oils in the white flowers, the rind, and the leaves.

Two plants in particular have been found to affect mood and state of mind and therefore can be used as a form of relaxation therapy. A study at the University of Miami Medical School found that people who inhaled the scent of lavender or rosemary were less anxious and more relaxed. Participants in the lavender group experienced an increase in beta band activity (suggesting drowsiness), an improvement in mood, and a feeling of greater relaxation. The rosemary group showed a decrease in alpha and beta power, suggesting alertness and lower levels of anxiety.[11] Other oils with calming properties include chamomile, geranium, and neroli.

> *One study found that people who inhaled the scent of lavender or rosemary were less anxious and more relaxed.*

Because it is safe and inexpensive, you might want to make aromatherapy a part of your relaxation regimen. According to Myra Cameron, author of *Mother Nature's Guide to Vibrant Beauty and Health*, you can practice this technique in three ways: through inhalation, water therapy, or massage. She explains, "Whether in mist or liquid form, essential oils are able to penetrate easily through the skin due to their small molecules. This sounds surprising because usually oils have large molecules that sit on the surface of the skin. But essential oils do not have an oily texture. These oils are called 'volatile' liquids because they evaporate when exposed to the air. They feel as light to the touch as water or alcohol. They disappear almost instantly when applied to the skin."[12]

Say a Little Prayer

Some find that prayer can have relaxing benefits similar to those of meditation. If you are spiritually inclined, a daily prayer session gives you quiet downtime. You might repeat the same prayer over and over to let your body relax into the rhythm of the words. In your petitions for fertility, you may find peace and acceptance. You also may find a miracle.

That's what happened when researchers at Columbia University found that women at an in vitro fertilization clinic in Korea had higher pregnancy rates when, unknown to the patients, total strangers were asked to pray for their success. The study involved 199 women who went to Cha Hospital for infertility treatments. None knew about the prayer study, and the medical staff caring for them also was unaware of it. The researchers gave members of different Christian denominations in the United States, Canada, and Australians photographs of the patients and asked them to pray. The women who were prayed for had a 50 percent pregnancy rate, compared with a 26 percent rate for the women not prayed for.

The lead author of this study, Dr. Rogerio A. Lobo, Columbia's chairman of obstetrics and gynecology, said he was initially unwilling to publish the results because they seemed so improbable. But they could not be ignored. "It was not even something that was borderline significant," Dr. Lobo said. "It was highly significant."[13]

Say Nice Things to Yourself

Many therapists use what's called *cognitive restructuring* to help couples deal with the negative aspects of infertility. This technique is not hard to do, and you can try it yourself at home.

Cognitive restructuring focuses on negative and noncoping thoughts caused by experiences such as disappointment, low self-esteem, guilt, embarrassment, and repeated treatment failures. Have you ever said to yourself statements such as, "I'll never get pregnant," "This is all my fault," "God is punishing me," or "I don't deserve to have a child"? These voices in your head contribute to stress and depression and make being infertile far more difficult than it needs to be. That's where cognitive restructuring can help. It teaches you to challenge those thoughts and gain greater control over what you think and therefore how you feel. It teaches you that you are not a hapless victim.

Cognitive restructuring teaches you that you are not a hapless victim.

Alice Domar, Ph.D., who directs the women's health programs at Harvard Medical School's world-renowned Division of Behavioral Medicine, has had much success with cognitive restructuring. "At its best," says Dr. Domar, "cognitive restructuring fosters a realistic optimism, in which we grapple with hard realities at the same time that we cultivate kindness toward ourselves." Women who join Dr. Domar's Behavioral Medicine Program for Infertility are taught how to uncover negative thoughts and check to see where those thoughts come from and whether they're valid. They are also coached in how to discover the reality of their situations and to replace their nasty mental tapes with more truthful and compassionate messages. They learn that the purpose of challenging negative thoughts is to confront the thought honestly, figure out its source and look at its effect on you, and then put it to the test of logic.

You can try this approach, too, by asking yourself the following four questions recommended by Dr. Domar the very next time you say something unkind to yourself:

1. Does this thought contribute to my stress?
2. Where did I learn this thought?
3. Is this thought logical?
4. Is this thought true?

When you practice cognitive restructuring on your own, Dr. Domar suggests that it might help to write down your negative thoughts and answers to the four questions. "Some of my patients," she says, "keep a literal 'diary of distortions,' in which they write down their automatic negative thoughts every day. The records they keep are powerful testimony to how much suffering is caused by mental trickery. They also use the diaries to challenge and restructure these thoughts, writing down their new thoughts and reminding themselves to live by them." You can learn more about Dr. Domar's Harvard Behavioral Medicine Program for Infertility in her book, *Healing Mind, Healthy Woman* (Holt, 1996).

Starting today, listen to what you say to yourself. Stop the thought immediately if you hear yourself getting wrapped up in any of these negative patterns:

- **Catastrophizing:** "My life is ruined."
- **Overgeneralizing:** "This will never end."
- **Personalizing:** "Leave it to me to be infertile."
- **Obsessing:** "This is awful. This is terrible. I can't stand this."

After you analyze these kinds of thoughts with the four questions recommended earlier, replace them with positive, kind, and loving thoughts. Make a habit of making statements like these:

- "It takes a courageous person to live through this."
- "I love and believe in myself."
- "I'm learning how to take control of my life."
- "I accept myself the way I am and will make the best of this life I have."
- "I am a good person."

> *When you learn to change the way you think about infertility, you will also learn that infertility does not define who you are as a person.*

With some persistence and practice, you can lean to identify your negative thoughts, challenge them, and replace them with more appropriate and loving thoughts. When you learn to change the way you think about infertility, you will also learn that infertility does not define who you are as a person.

Practice Yoga

The word *yoga* means "to join or yoke together" because it brings the body and mind together into one harmonious experience. In ancient times, the desire for greater personal freedom, health and long life, and heightened self-understanding gave birth to this system of physical and mental exercise, which has since spread throughout the world. The exercises of yoga are designed to put pressure on the glandular systems of the body, thereby increasing its efficiency and total health.[14]

You can also use many of the yoga poses to attain a state of relaxation and peace of mind.

Anna Delury, B.S., from Los Angeles, California, practices and teaches yoga in the tradition of B. K. S. Iyengar and specializes in pre- and post-natal yoga classes. Due to her own experience with infertility, Delury understands the complete emotional devastation that can accompany the diagnosis and treatment of infertility, and she knows personally how yoga can give you back your life again. "Yoga," she says, "works not only on releasing the stress on the musculoskeletal system of the body but also on the other systems of the body: the endocrine system, the immune system, the organic, the respiratory, and circulatory systems are all relieved of the burden of stress through yoga."

Sample Yoga Poses

Although many yoga poses are complex and require guidance by a professional yoga teacher, you can try some basic poses at home to get you started. Delury recommends the following three poses to ease stress and tension. If you do them every day in the order they are listed, you'll find the 5 to 10 minutes you dedicate to daily yoga will reward you with an instant feeling of calm.

To get the most out of these poses, Delury offers these tips:

- You can do these poses at any time of day, but you should do them on an empty stomach (3 to 4 hours after a large meal).
- Wear comfortable clothing.
- Avoid cold or drafty places when practicing your poses.
- Do not do these poses without professional guidance if you are pregnant and have a history of miscarriage or have lower back ailments.

Pose 1: Uttanasana. (See figure 6.1.) Stand with your feet about 12 inches apart. Grab each elbow with the opposite hand and bring your

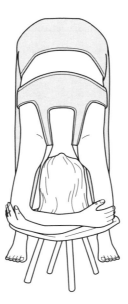

Figure 6.1—*Uttanasana*

arms over the head. Exhale and bend over. Rest your head on a pillow you've placed on a table or chair in front of you. If you are more flexible and can bend farther down, rest your head on a stack of books or blocks placed on the floor. Relax the head and breathe evenly. Stay in this position for 1 to 3 minutes. Inhale and come back up, bringing your legs together.

Pose 2: Baddhakonasana. (See figure 6.2.) Sit with a straight back against a wall on one or two folded blankets that give your body an upward lift in the torso. Bend your knees and drop each to its respective side. Bring your feet together and line them up with the soles touching. Bring the heels as close as possible to the pubis. Hold your toes or ankles. Stretch your thighs by bringing your knees down to the floor as far as possible. Stretch your trunk up and open the chest. Keep your head level. Hold this pose for 1 minute.

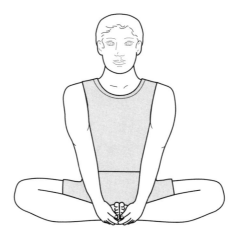

Figure 6.2—*Baddhakonasana*

Pose 3: Supta Baddhakonasana. (See figure 6.3.) This pose is done with a bolster (a folded blanket or pillows will do) as a backrest and a folded towel as a headrest. In a sitting position, bring the soles of your feet together with your knees apart. Place a support like a rolled-up towel or a phone book under each knee to ease any pressure. Use a strap (or a belt or necktie) to keep your feet together and a nonslip rubber mat to keep them from sliding away from the body. Lie back

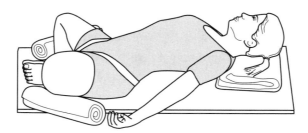

Figure 6.3—*Supta Baddhakonasana*

on the bolster, letting your arms fall comfortably to your sides. Hold this pose for 5 to 10 minutes.

Yoga for Infertility

Some say that yoga can restore fertility, and in some cases this may be true. During the stress response, the body releases epinephrine, which constricts blood vessels. This constriction may occur in the uterus, thus interfering with conception. According to a recent article published in *Yoga Journal*, this reaction coincides with the yogic idea of *apana*, the downward-moving energy that for women is centered in the pelvis. "Allowing apana to flow freely," says author Judith Hanson Lasater, "could be the key for reproduction to occur. There are some yoga poses that help to gently stimulate apana energy, as well as increase micro-circulation in the reproductive tract."[15]

> *Anything you find that leads you to a relaxed state will improve the overall quality of your life.*

You might want to take a look at some of these poses as they are discussed and illustrated in the book, *Yoga: A Path to Holistic Health*, by B. K. S. Iyengar (DK Publishing, 2001). But because infertility is a highly individualized life state with many varied causes, it is best to find a certified instructor experienced in working with infertile couples to guide you.

More Ways to Relax

When you're comfortable with the basics we've considered thus far, go on to explore other types of relaxation strategies. There is no strategy created specifically for infertility; anything you find that leads you to a relaxed state will improve the overall quality of your life. You can find various types of relaxation programs on the bookshelves, for example. (The classic in this field is Dr. Herbert Benson's *The Relaxation Response*.) You can buy relaxation audios and videotapes that take you through the steps of various exercises. Or consider enrolling in a class about more advanced types of relaxation techniques that may require some guidance and supervision to use them effectively, such as advanced yoga, hypnosis, and meditation.

THE INFERTILITY–DEPRESSION LINK

You probably won't be surprised to hear that there is a link between depression and infertility. After all, through this experience, your relationships, your sex life, your finances, and your image of who you are and where you're going all can be thrown into turmoil. In her book, *Six Steps to Increased Infertility*, Dr. Domar states that the depression scores of infertile women are very much like those of women who have cancer, heart disease, or HIV. "Almost 11 percent of infertile women meet the psychological criteria for a current, major depressive episode," she says. "Infertile women usually state that infertility is the worst crisis of their lives, that it's even worse than divorce or the death of a parent."

In one study, for example, Dr. Domar points out that women with a history of depression were nearly twice as likely to experience infertility as women who didn't have such a history. In other research, she says women who already had several cycles of IVF treatment and were depressed before continuing it had a 13 percent pregnancy rate. Women who weren't depressed before receiving IVF had a 29 percent rate of conception.[16]

> *In one study, women with a history of depression were nearly twice as likely to experience infertility as women who didn't have such a history.*

Given this link between depression and fertility, it is smart to examine your state of emotional health before continuing your efforts to conceive. To recognize and then do something about depression, you need to be able to identify its symptoms.

Keep in mind that depression isn't the same as sadness or a sense of feeling down or anxious. We all have those feelings at different times throughout our lives. True depression makes it almost impossible to carry on usual activities, sleep, eat, or enjoy life. Pleasure seems a thing of the past. The National Institutes of Mental Health say that if you have experienced four or more of the following symptoms for more than 2 weeks, you are at risk for clinical depression and should have a physical and psychological evaluation by a medical physician:

- A persistent sad, anxious, or "empty" mood

- Loss of interest or pleasure in ordinary activities, including sex

- Sleep problems (insomnia, oversleeping, early-morning waking)

- Eating problems (loss of appetite or weight, weight gain)

- Difficulty concentrating, remembering, or making decisions

- Feelings of hopelessness or pessimism

Resource Referral

Find out more about depression by contacting these organizations:

National Foundation for Depressive Illness
P.O. Box 2257
New York, NY 10116
Phone: (800) 239-1265
Web site: www.depression.org

National Mental Health Association
1021 Prince Street
Alexandria, VA 22314
Phone: (800) 969-6642
Web site: www.nmha.org

- Feelings of guilt, worthlessness, or helplessness

- Thoughts of death or suicide; a suicide attempt

- Irritability

- Excessive crying

- Recurring aches and pains that don't respond to treatment[17]

PROFESSIONAL COUNSELING

When faced with the fact of infertility, emotions run high, tempers are often short, and guilt frequently runs rampant. What to do? In these circumstances, some infertile couples readily seek professional counseling. When they see that their infertility is affecting the way they think about themselves, their partners, and their lives, they reach out for help in coping with their negative feelings. Other couples, however, view infertility as a purely physical problem, not a psychological one. With good reason, they may resent the implication that their infertility is their own fault caused by a mental weakness (e.g., being too stressed or too obsessed) and don't see the point of talking to a counselor. Others are just too focused on the time, effort, and cost of medical procedures to even think about adding one more appointment to their calendar. If you are one of these people avoiding counseling, you might want to rethink that decision.

If you are one of these people avoiding counseling, you might want to rethink that decision.

Jane Rosenthal, M.D., who is an assistant professor of psychiatry at Columbia Presbyterian Medical Center in New York City and a psychotherapist working with infertile couples, has seen how professional counseling can help enrich lives torn by infertility. "I absolutely believe that infertile couples can benefit from professional counseling," she says. "For most people, this is an unexpected life event that comes as a huge shock with psychological repercussions. This is why it is very useful for the couple to have the opportunity to take a look at the impact this has had on their life and the way it has affected their relationship, their finances, and their self-image. These are things that some couples just can't talk about together, so it's useful to have someone who has had experience working with infertile couples to help them talk about how they view the experience and issues like fairness ('Why this is happening to us?') and resentment ('Whose fault is this?')."

In addition, a complicated self-esteem issue often gets ignored in the process of infertility work. "It's very hard to understand why the body isn't working the way it's supposed to and the way you expected it to," says Dr. Rosenthal. "This is a time that challenges one's assumptions about things that are supposed to be automatic in one's lifetime. It's also a situation in which you have to answer questions that go unasked in other people's lives. Most people don't have to ask themselves why they want to be parents, and yet that is the kind of question that people need to ask themselves when they begin rearranging their lives to accommodate infertility treatments or when they're facing depression over a decision to remain childless. These kind of internal challenges are hard to face, and the answers to these questions that seem so unfair are hard to verbalize. It is painful, but useful, to put this into words."

If you decide to see a therapist, look for one who has experience working with infertile couples.

If you decide to see a therapist, look for one who has experience working with infertile couples. These are people who understand what you're feeling and have knowledge about the medical procedures you may be going through. It's best to find a therapist through personal referrals from trusted friends or physicians, but you can also find a list of therapists who specialize in infertility on the RESOLVE Web site at www.resolve.org.

There is no doubt that infertility is not solely a physical problem. It can directly affect a person's mental and emotional health, which in some cases has been known to create a vicious cycle that further decreases the likelihood of conception. For this reason, it is very important to make an effort to keep your mind and spirit calm during this difficult time and look to the future with hope. The following chapter will give you a glimpse at where the future of infertility treatment is headed and how you may benefit from these exciting new possibilities.

CHAPTER 7

A Future Wrapped in High Hopes and Controversy

ASK YOUR GRANDMOTHER how the medical community treated the common cold when she was a young woman, and you'll find that today's recommended remedy of rest and fluids is the same prescription given in her day also. Then ask her what the treatment was for infertility, and she'll probably offer no more than a shoulder shrug. This response will give you an idea of how, in the span of two generations, advances in the field of human reproduction have exploded. While reproductive endocrinologists are far from having all the answers, they have more to offer the infertile couple today than at any other time in history. Every day children are born to people who, in the past, would never have been biological parents, which is a gift of incalculable measure.

The number of couples and individuals benefiting from improvements in assisted reproductive technologies continues to grow at significant rates. According to the statistics released in 2002 by the Centers for Disease Control and Prevention, fertility procedures in the United States jumped by 27 percent in just 2 years. The number of procedures rose from 64,724 in 1996 to 81,899 in 1998. (These numbers do not include artificial insemination.) The number of clinics offering these services also increased, growing from about 40 in vitro fertilization clinics in 1986 to over 370 today.[1]

Still, there is much room for improvement. Of those nearly 82,000 procedures in 1998, only about 20,000 led to live births.[2] For this reason, researchers continue their search for more answers to the questions surrounding infertility. They often find that for every two steps forward, they must take one step back because working with live embryos in a research environment raises many ethical, moral, social, and financial issues that must be addressed as the future of assisted human reproduction continues to advance.

> **West Coast Babies**
>
> According to the Centers for Disease Control (CDC), California led the nation with 10,615 fertility procedures in 1998. The CDC said none were performed in Alaska, Idaho, Maine, and Montana because there were no clinics in those states.[3]

This chapter discusses some of the most promising areas of research and offers a look at the controversies surrounding many of the proposed procedures and possibilities. It does not offer answers to the debate, but rather an honest look at the questions.

ADVANCES IN ASSISTED REPRODUCTIVE TECHNOLOGY (ART)

It's quite impressive that medical technology has advanced to the point where it can take a woman's egg, combine it in a petri dish with a man's sperm, and create a fertilized embryo that can then be transferred into the female, where it will grow into a healthy baby. Although we still have much to learn about this process before total success can be claimed, each day medical researchers are taking small steps forward to improve your chances of having your baby.

Until recently, only about 10 percent of all embryos survived the transfer back into the uterus.[4] Success rates were particularly poor for women over age 38. Now, newer pretransfer procedures are being performed in select clinics across the country that are giving many women renewed hope. These procedures include assisted hatching, fragment removal, blastocyst culture and transfer, preimplantation diagnosis, and cytoplasmic transfer.

Assisted Hatching

When embryos are transferred into the uterus, they are covered with an outer coating known as the *zona pellucida*. This coating must dissolve so the embryo can "hatch" and attach itself to the uterine wall. If a woman has had repeated IVF failures at this point, the doctor can use a microscopic glass tube to place a minute amount of a dissolving fluid on the outer coating of the embryo. There is a minimal risk that the embryo may be damaged through this technique, but doctors offering assisted hatching feel the benefits outweigh the risks for women with repeat failures. Contemporary management recommends this procedure for older women and those with prior failures as long as the clinic has competent lab personnel to perform this technique.

Doctors offering assisted hatching feel the benefits outweigh the risks for women with repeat IVF failures.

Fragment Removal

Fragments are little pieces of cells that are left behind when embryos divide inefficiently. Jacques Cohen, Ph.D., scientific director of the Institute for Reproductive Medicine and Science at Saint Barnabas Medical Center in Livingston, New Jersey, says, "Normally, fragments are not a hindrance to further development and pregnancy because they occur in about 85 percent of all embryos. But when there are a lot of them, it interferes with normal development." Dr. Cohen pierces the shells of these fertilized eggs and removes their fragments. This procedure is now being evaluated in many IVF clinics in the hope of boosting a poor-quality embryo's chance of implanting.[5]

Paul Gindoff, M.D., director at George Washington University Medical Center's IVF unit, tempers this enthusiasm: "We have all had the clinical experience of patients having not only normal singleton pregnancies with fragmented embryos but even multiple pregnancies. Clearly, the cause and effect among embryo quality, fragmentation, and implantation are not fully understood."

Blastocyst Culture and Transfer

During an IVF procedure, the egg and sperm are placed in a culture medium to fertilize. In the past, a four-celled embryo was transferred to the woman's uterus 48 hours after fertilization. As laboratory techniques improved, the embryos were kept in the medium for 3 days before transfer where they would grow to 8- to 10-cell embryos. Now it is possible to keep the embryos in the culture medium up to 5 days before transfer. This 5-day-old embryo is called a *blastocyst* and has divided into hundreds of cells.

Mark Perloe, M.D., medical director at Georgia Reproductive Specialists and a clinical assistant professor in obstetrics and gynecology at the Medical College of Georgia, believes that blastocyst transfer holds important possibilities for the future success of IVF procedures. "As time and culture media improved," says Dr. Perloe, "we found we could come up with specific media data at each stage during the growth cycle. We found that the needs of a fertilized egg on day 2 were different from the needs on day 3 or 4. So, by making a culture media to meet the needs of the embryo at each time period, we have been able to grow these embryos for 5 days before transfer."

Blastocyst transfer is an exciting advance in assisted reproductive technology because it allows doctors to better evaluate the health and viability of the embryos before transfer. "A good portion of embryos that appear healthy on the third day will not make it to the fifth day," cautions Dr. Perloe. "I believe this is because the embryos that die between the third and fifth day are inherently unhealthy. In the first 2 to 3 days, the growth of the embryo is predominantly dependent on enzymes and proteins in the egg from the mother. It's only on the fourth or fifth day that the growth requires the genetic contribution from both father and mother to continue development. So the embryo could develop normally and look very good on the third day because the mother's egg contained normal chromosomes. But the quality of the sperm contribution will not be known until the fourth or fifth day. Therefore, the further out the transfer can be done, the more likely the selected embryos are to be genetically normal and viable. When this is the case, there tends to be a higher rate of successful implantation, and as an added benefit, fewer embryos can be transferred, reducing the risk of higher-order multiples."

> *Blastocyst transfer is an exciting advance in assisted reproductive technology because it allows doctors to better evaluate the health and viability of the embryos before transfer.*

Despite the advantages of a blastocyst transfer, waiting 5 days is not routine and still a bit controversial. Dr. Perloe explains: "As embryos develop, each day their needs become more demanding. Not all laboratories have the conditions or culture medium necessary to optimally grow embryos for 5 days. In most cases where blastocyst transfer is possible, the decision is not made until the physician evaluates the embryos' health on day 3 and determines whether he or she thinks they have a good chance to make it to blastocyst.

"The future goal in this area is to determine the point in time at which an embryo is better off growing inside the uterus than in the laboratory," he continues. "The hope is to optimize the culture environment so we can grow the embryos longer and better choose which ones to transfer, and use a fewer number of transfers. Of course, this brings up the issue of safety versus success rates. Will we work to transfer healthier but fewer embryos even if that results in a lower pregnancy rate? This will be an ongoing debate as the ability to nurture embryos outside the womb for longer periods increases."

In a study published in 2000, Dr. Gindoff's group at George Washington University Medical Center showed that blastocyst transfer was able to help women with prior IVF failures who had previously only had day-3 eight-cell embryo transfers. "The results of our study were very exciting," says Dr. Gindoff, "allowing a second-line treatment for many women after IVF failure."

Preimplantation Diagnosis

If you opt for in vitro fertilization, you may soon have the opportunity to pick and choose only the healthiest embryos for transfer through a process call *preimplantation genetic diagnosis* (PGD). The American Society for Reproductive Medicine (ASRM) tells us that PGD is a technique that can be used during IVF procedures to test embryos for genetic disorders prior to their transfer to the uterus. This technologically advanced diagnostic procedure makes it possible for couples with serious inherited genetic disorders to decrease the risk of having a child who is affected the same way. The procedure is currently available in a few selected fertility clinics throughout the country.

This technologically advanced diagnostic procedure makes it possible for couples with serious inherited genetic disorders to decrease the risk of having a child who is affected the same way.

Not all genetic disorders can be identified in embryos with this technique, but the ASRM lists the following disorders that PGD can detect at this time:

a-1-antitrypsin deficiency
Charcot-Marie-Tooth disease
cystic fibrosis
Down's syndrome
Duchenne muscular dystrophy
fragile X syndrome

hemophilia A
Lesch–Nyhan syndrome
Retinitis pigmentosa
Tay-Sachs disease
Turner's syndrome[6]

It is also believed that PGD may lead to improved chances of successful pregnancy for older women and for those who have had repeat miscarriages. The primary reason that the chance of pregnancy diminishes with age is the increased incidence of chromosomal abnormalities in the egg. More frequently in women over age 35, the egg has one extra or one missing chromosome, resulting in embryo death and infertility, spontaneous abortions, or babies with Down's syndrome or other chromosomal abnormalities.

By examining chromosomal abnormalities before implantation, researchers at Saint Barnabas Medical Center have found significant reduction in the rate of miscarriage from 23 percent to 9 percent. In women who experienced repeated miscarriages, the rate went from 100 percent to only 15 percent.[7] These impressive results occur because PGD can identify compromised embryos, allowing the physician to better determine which embryos should be transferred.

The PGD and Controversy

Up to this point, PGD has been reserved almost exclusively for couples at risk for having babies with certain genetic diseases. However, it has always been clear that the method could easily be used for other purposes. This possibility is what

> *It is also believed that PGD may lead to improved chances of successful pregnancy for older women and for those who have had repeat miscarriages.*

makes it controversial. Some fear that the ability to choose only select embryos is a short throw away from fast-ordering any number of genetic traits—and discarding those we don't like. The hot debate right now is over sex selection through PGD.

It is quite simple for an embryologist to see whether the embryo is male, with an X and a Y chromosome, or female, with two X chromosomes. So why not choose the sex of your baby? For example, if you are having an IVF procedure and plan to have only one child and would like it to be a male to carry on the family name, why not ask the doctor to select only male embryos for transfer to the uterus? If you already have a boy, why not now ask for a girl? As simple as the request may seem, this use of PGD poses ethical questions.

In a detailed ethics report in 1999, the ASRM said that selecting and implanting embryos of a particular sex solely for the purpose of guaranteeing parents that their child would be a boy or a girl "should be discouraged" because of serious ethical concerns. But then in May 2001, the Ethics Committee of the ASRM released a new position on gender selection that reads:

Physicians should be free to offer preconception gender selection in clinical settings to couples who are seeking gender variety in their offspring if the couples (1) are fully informed of the risks of failure, (2) affirm that they will fully accept children of the opposite sex if the preconception gender selection fails, (3) are counseled about having unrealistic expectations about the behavior of children of the preferred gender, and (4) are offered the opportunity to participate in research to track and access the safety, efficacy, and demographics of preconception gender selection.[8]

This report has raised controversy among ASRM members, and not all practitioners honor requests for gender selection during IVF procedures. "Sex selection is sex discrimination, and I don't think that is ethical," says James Grifo, M.D., a reproductive endocrinologist at New York University Medical Center.[9] Others voice concerns that gender selection can upset the natural balance between men and women in the population. Some worry that sex selection opens the door to embryo selection based on eye color, height, intelligence, and so on.

> *The hot debate right now is over sex selection through PGD.*

Reproductive endocrinologists don't expect fertile couples to be beating down their door wanting IVF for sex selection purposes. But still the debate continues. The concern over widespread use of any kind of PGD comes down to the question of how common IVF, as opposed to sexual intercourse, becomes as a method of human reproduction.

Cytoplasmic Transfer

IVF procedures have given the precious gift of parenthood to thousands of infertile couples, but the present methods of IVF still fail many thousands more. Doctors at the Institute for Reproductive Medicine and Science at Saint Barnabas Hospital have found a way to help some of these couples, but the method has become the focus of great debate.

Dr. Cohen and Steen Willadsen, Ph.D., found that one group of women under age 40 who had repeated failed IVF cycles were able to achieve reasonable numbers of follicles when stimulated and had high estradiol levels, yet after successful fertilization with healthy sperm, they had poor subsequent embryo development and implantation success. When the embryologists saw that the eggs with normal chromosomes were not able to develop properly even under ideal conditions, Drs. Cohen and Willadsen realized that the reason may lie in the cytoplasm of the egg—the area within the shell of the egg that lies outside the nucleus, outside the region that contains the genetic material or DNA.

"The cytoplasm," says David Sable, M.D., Drs. Cohen and Willadsen's colleague and director of the division of reproductive endocrinology and infertility at Saint. Barnabas, "includes a myriad of components. One component is mitochondria. Remember the 'powerhouse' of the cell from high school biology? Mitochondria provide energy to the cell, fuel for many of its functions including, presumably, cell division, but lately have been found to be involved in many more crucial processes. If an egg has inadequate mitochondria, it seems logical that this would result in poor embryo formation. Other cytoplasmic factors are likely to play an important role as well."

Dr. Gindoff adds, "Mitochondria have their own separate genetic material—DNA. This is coding for important steps and mechanisms in early embryo division and possibly implantation."

> If the cause of the egg problem is in the cytoplasm, then why not replace just the cytoplasm with donated cytoplasm, rather than use an entire donated egg?

In the past, women in this situation were told that donor egg IVF or adoption were their only options for achieving parenthood. But Drs. Cohen, Sable, and their colleagues reasoned that if the cause of the egg problem is in the cytoplasm, then why not replace just the cytoplasm with donated cytoplasm, rather than use an entire donated egg, thus keeping the mother's own genetic contribution to the pregnancy? This was the premise on which they developed cytoplasmic transfer (also called *ooplasmic transfer*).

The controversy over this procedure developed when the researchers tested the blood of two of the resulting children at 1 year of age. Using genetic fingerprinting techniques, they found that some children had mitochondrial DNA from the donor egg. The headlines in both medical and lay media screamed the news of the first cases of "human germline genetic modification resulting in normal, healthy children." In other words, these children had DNA from three parents.

Dr. Sable feels the meaning of this finding has been misunderstood and has caused an overreaction in the medical community. "Yes," he freely admits, "the donated mitochondria do have their own DNA, but that DNA is virtually identical in every human being in the world except for a tiny area called the *hypervariable region*. This area is analogous to a license plate on a car. It has almost no function whatsoever. It is not a gene; it doesn't code for any products; it's a means of identifying where the mitochondria come from. In fact, there is a precedent for this in nature: The hypervariable region has been known to mutate on its own, and there are people who have different types of DNA in that region naturally. It doesn't seem to be associated with any dysfunction or disease."

The term genetic modification *is associated with altering DNA to modify inherited traits, which is prohibited by the Recombinant DNA Advisory Committee (RAC). Does cytoplasmic transfer violate this ban?*

Nonetheless, the controversy persists. The term *genetic modification* is associated with altering DNA to modify inherited traits, which is prohibited by the Recombinant DNA Advisory Committee (RAC). Does cytoplasmic transfer violate this ban? "No," says Dr. Sable. "No manipulation or modification of the donor's or recipient's nuclear or mitochondrial genome occurred, and no altered genes were transferred. The headlines that grabbed attention by talking about babies with three parents was, I believe, a sensationalized and willful misunderstanding of the science behind the procedure."

Because there is the issue of DNA from a third party, the Federal Drug Administration (FDA) has stopped all cytoplasmic transfers and has required the doctors at St. Barnabas and any others that have used

---

Scanning for Chromosomal Abnormalities

Doctors can now examine, to some degree, the genetic makeup of an IVF embryo by doing biopsies. "We can do quick scanning of the markers for up to eight different chromosomes, for example," says Dr. Mark Perloe, medical director at Georgia Reproductive Specialists, "to see if the embryo is missing a full chromosome or if it has an extra chromosome. This is not done on a routine basis because the test destroys the embryo, but this is where a lot of research is going. Researchers continue to look for other biochemical markers that will help evaluate the health of the embryo."

---

the experimental technique to apply for formal oversight and approval from the FDA. "Certainly we are going to comply with anything the FDA asks us to do," says Dr. Sable. He feels that when doctors started going inside the egg to manipulate fertilization, we entered a new world. "Cytoplasmic transfer," he says, "is a logical extension of the assisted reproductive technologies that have been developed so far. It is a valid, though experimental, treatment modality." Time will tell.

GOOD NEWS FOR MEN, TOO

The medical advances that offer hope for the improved treatment of infertility problems have not been confined only to women. The most basic diagnostic procedure for males is still a sperm analysis, but a new sperm analysis test can more quickly pick up chromosomal problems in sperm before they are used in IUI or IVF procedures.

"When we do a semen analysis," says Dr. Perloe, "it's like going to the UPS Web site with a tracking number. You can find out when your package is going to arrive and if the box has become damaged. But you can't determine if what's inside the box is really what you ordered or if it is of good quality. Sperm is like a little UPS delivery truck, and sperm analysis of the past was like that tracking system that could tell us that the sperm were delivering chromosomes and DNA, but we couldn't find out anything about their quality.

"Now we have a tracking system that can evaluate the overall quality of the DNA inside the male's sperm," Dr. Perloe explains. "The new sperm chromatin structure assay (SCSA) test can pick up the percentage of sperm with DNA damage caused by things like cigarette smoking, hot tubbing, and a lot of times even exposure to environmental toxins. If more than 30 percent of the sperm have these DNA breaks, IVF success rates plummet."

> *A new sperm analysis test can more quickly pick up chromosomal problems in sperm before they are used in IUI or IVF procedures.*

Four common problem areas stand out. One reason for male factor infertility is that the brain may not be sending the message to the testicle to make sperm. Only 3 to 4 percent of male infertility is caused in this way, but we are increasingly improving the protocols for stimulating the testicle to generate adequate sperm. This condition is basically due to a hormonal imbalance.

A second reason for male factor infertility is that the testicle might not be responding to the message from the brain to make sperm due to some kind of chromosomal abnormality. In the journal *Proceedings of the National Academy of Sciences*, Japanese researcher Mito Kanatsu-Shinohara and his colleagues report that gene therapy may be useful in treating this kind of male infertility. They were specifically looking at a genetic cause of infertility in male mice that renders them unable to produce mature, functioning sperm. Gene therapy usually uses a harmless virus that is equipped with a normal copy of the defective gene. The normal copy of the gene should replace the abnormal one and restore function. The researchers injected the virus-gene combination into the male mice. Giving the normal copy of the gene restored the mice's ability to produce mature sperm. The researchers believe that the success of this procedure in male mice offers a promising treatment for infertility in men whose problems have a genetic cause.[10] However, we are many steps away from attempting this technique in humans.

Another reason for male factor infertility is outflow obstruction. In this case, physicians can now biopsy the testicle to get sperm out and unite with an egg through insemination or IVF (see chapter 4 for the details), or the obstruction can be surgically corrected.

Unexplained infertility, the fourth most common reason for male factor infertility, represents the majority of such cases. Studies are under way to correlate SCSA results with men who otherwise have normal semen parameters. However, abnormal SCSA results still do not preclude fertility or normalcy of offspring. Clinical use of these results remains controversial.

> *Gene therapy usually uses a harmless virus that is equipped with a normal copy of the defective gene.*

DEALING WITH THE PROBLEM OF HIGHER-ORDER MULTIPLES

Most members of the reproductive care medical community were not handing out cigars the day septuplets were born at Georgetown University Hospital in 2001. Higher-order multiples, as infants are called when they come in threes or more, are viewed as a medical failure— or even disaster. These multiple births are not the result of natural procreation; in almost all cases, they are caused by the use of fertility drugs such as clomiphene citrate or, more likely, gonadotropins and ART procedures such as controlled ovarian hyperstimulation with intrauterine insemination or IVF.

Having higher-order multiples is one instance where more is not better. The ASRM cautions that many medical complications ensue with multiples: "Fetal risks of multiple gestation include an increased chance of miscarriage, birth defects, premature birth, and the mental and/or physical problems that can result from premature delivery."[11] Premature birth is a major concern because multiples are routinely

---

Astounding Numbers

The National Center for Health Statistics (NCHS) reported that from 1980 through 1997, the annual number of twin births rose 52 percent (from 68,339 to 104,137), while the annual number of triplet and other higher-order multiple gestations rose over 400 percent (from 1,377 to 6,737).[12]

---

delivered early. The ASRM reports that the average length of pregnancy is 39 weeks for a single gestation, 35 weeks for twins, 33 weeks for triplets, and 29 weeks for quadruplets.

The mother also faces risks during a multiple gestation. These complications include pregnancy-induced high blood pressure, or preeclampsia (toxemia); diabetes; and vaginal/uterine hemorrhage.[13] Obviously, higher-order multiples are not a desirable outcome for any couple.

Because higher-order multiples complicate an ART conception, pregnancy, and delivery, physicians and researchers are looking for techniques and procedures that will reduce their likelihood when a couple has ovulation induction (OI) with intrauterine insemination (IUI) or an IVF procedure. Possible reduction strategies discussed here include practicing pregnancy reduction, performing fewer OIs with IUIs, rethinking clinic success rates, pushing for insurance reform, and including more patient education in infertility programs.

Pregnancy Reduction

When a couple finds that the woman is carrying higher-order multiples, they may be asked to consider the elimination of one or more of the fetuses. In this outpatient procedure, usually performed between 9 and 12 weeks' gestation (but sometimes as late as 24 weeks' gestation), a needle guided by ultrasound through either the abdomen or vagina injects potassium chloride into the embryonic heart. This fetus will then shortly die in utero and may be reabsorbed by the body.

Reducing the number of fetuses improves the chances of healthy survival for the remaining ones. However, for couples who have invested much time, money, and energy in trying to have children, this is a very painful decision. In addition to the fact that this procedure is prohibited by some religious beliefs, there is the dreadful possibility that all the embryos will expire. Every-one in the reproductive health care community agrees that dealing with higher-order multiples after the fact is the least desirable way to avoid this complication of ART.

> *Reducing the number of fetuses improves the chances of healthy survival for the remaining ones.*

Fewer Ovulation Inductions with Intrauterine Inseminations

Higher-order multiples are a side effect of advanced reproductive procedures, but they are far more common after OI with IUIs than with ART (generally IVF). A recent review of research literature published between 1990 and 1996 found that OI accounted for 10 to 69 percent of triplet gestations, compared to 24 to 30 percent from ART and 7 to 18 percent from spontaneous conceptions. OI accounted for 50 to 72 percent of higher-order multiple gestations, ART accounted for 42 percent of these births, and 6 to 7 percent of these gestations were from spontaneous conception.[14]

For this reason, reproductive endocrinologists such as James Madden, M.D., medical director of the Assisted Reproductive Technology Services Program at Presbyterian Hospital of Dallas, believe that OI/IUI will be phased out in favor of IVF. "We're in a time of transition," says Dr. Madden. "Five years ago you had to fail the OI/IUI in order to get to the IVF. But now there is more of a feeling that ovulation induction and IUI have an unacceptable absence of control—we can't dictate how many eggs will be fertilized. IVF gives much better control because we can select only one or two quality embryos for transfer, significantly reducing the number of multiple births."

The physician who uses OI/IUI has a strong role to play in how often this procedure results in higher-order multiples. According to Dr. Madden, "A physician cannot be afraid to tell a couple that there are too many follicles (eggs), and so the cycle has to be canceled, and they have to sleep in separate bedrooms for a while. The couple may cry and sometimes will angrily leave the practice. But we have to accept these things because we have a moral obligation not to put women at risk for having three or four babies.

> *IVF gives much better control [than OI/IUI] because we can select only one or two quality embryos for transfer, significantly reducing the number of multiple births.*
>
> *—JAMES MADDEN, M.D.*

Dr. Madden adds, "This whole scenario can be avoided by using IVF with the transfer of one or two embryos. We have to learn that getting pregnant is not the ultimate goal. The goal is to give birth to a healthy child."

Blastocyst Transfer

As you'll recall from the earlier discussion in this chapter, a blastocyst is a 5-day-old embryo that has divided into hundreds of cells. Blastocyst transfer seems to improve IVF pregnancy rates because it allows doctors to better evaluate the health and viability of the embryos, allowing them to choose only the healthiest for transfer. As an added bonus, blastocyst transfer also allows doctors to transfer fewer embryos without reducing the chances of pregnancy. A Washington, D.C.–based team, led by Dr. Gindoff, found that for women with good prognosis, blastocyst transfer lowered the multiple pregnancy rate without lowering overall pregnancy rates. Similarly, a team from New York University found that in their donor egg program, reducing the number of blastocyst embryos transferred from three to two reduced the triplet pregnancy rate without reducing the overall pregnancy rate.[15] Findings like these are encouraging many ART physicians to move toward blastocyst transfer whenever possible.

Clinic Success Rates

Competition among fertility clinics is one of the reasons for continued multiple gestations despite the increasing knowledge about how to lower their occurrence. When choosing a fertility clinic, many couples investigate its success rate. This figure, available in the clinic's brochure, on its Web site, and through the Centers for Disease Control, indicates what percentage of infertile couples who come to the clinic deliver a living child. It is no secret that to keep those numbers up, some physicians ignore the ASRM's recommendation to transfer only two to four embryos at a time, depending on the woman's age and prognosis. In other cases, once a multiple gestation has been obtained, the patient may be encouraged to undergo selective reduction, leading to a singleton or twin delivery. Thus, the real occurrence of multiple implantations is camouflaged and hidden by aggressive management.

> Competition among fertility clinics is one of the reasons for continued multiple gestations despite the increasing knowledge about how to lower their occurrence.

Many in the medical community agree with Dr. Madden, who sees this occurrence as a troubling sign. "If clinicians should ever think that their success rates are more relevant than the quality of life of the offspring," he says, "that's going to lead to the transfer of more embryos and more multiple gestations. Once any medical procedure gets out of the hands of doctors who put the rights and needs of their patients first and into the hands of industry, then you have considerations like supply and demand, marketing plans, and balance sheets to worry about." Many fine and competent doctors believe that although ART is high-tech, it is still medicine and should stay that way.

Insurance Reform

Insurance companies get blamed for a lot of things, but are they really the cause of the continued high rates of multiple gestations? Yes, say many in the know. It's only logical that if your policy does not cover infertility treatments, you're not going to want to cancel an OI/IUI cycle because you have too many eggs when you're paying out of your own pocket. Also, if you're paying for an IVF procedure, you're not going to want to risk transferring only one embryo when your chances of a pregnancy are better when transferring five. Basically, economics influence the choices some couples are forced to make.

> *B*asically, economics influence the choices some couples are forced to make.

Even those with insurance coverage face the kinds of decisions that lead to higher-order multiples due to limits on that coverage. "If a provider offers, let's say, a $10,000 lifetime benefit for assisted reproduction," explains Dr. Madden, "many couples will decide to try assisted reproductive technology just once. In this circumstance, they are a bit more inclined to separate themselves from their own good judgment. So on the IVF transfer day, the doctor may say, 'We'd like to transfer only one embryo because it looks so good.' The couple may say, 'No way. This is our only chance at this, and we don't want to hear anything that sounds like it will reduce our chances of getting pregnant.' These couples can't help but think that three babies would be better than none. In our practice, the couple has the last word, and so even when we want to do the right thing to reduce multiple gestations, sometimes that's not what happens because of the money involved."

Many believe the insurance companies could influence a reduction in multiple embryo transfers by offering coverage to all subscribers in all states. Margaret Hollister, executive director of RESOLVE, says, "It has been shown that in states with mandated insurance coverage for infertility treatment, both health-care costs and the number of multiple births are significantly reduced."[16] The insurance companies may also affect a reduction in multiple births by changing their payout plans when they do offer coverage. Talks are under way focusing on the possibility of paying physicians more for fertility treatments leading to the delivery of a single baby. Certainly the up-front costs would be far less than the cost of caring for multiple birth babies.

Patient Education

Dr. Madden believes that the key to reducing higher-order multiples lies in patient education. "We have to help people think through the process. They need to understand the difficulties involved in a multiple gestation—not just in the pregnancy, but in the problems the offspring might have. We know there will be a day of transfer (for us that's usually on the fifth day), and at that time we'll discuss with the patient what the embryos look like and what the likelihood is that they will become babies. Routinely, we transfer two embryos, but in selected instances when a blastocyst looks superlative, we would suggest a single embryo transfer to mimic as closely as possible what ordinarily happens in spontaneous conception.

"If you spring the idea of transferring only one embryo on people at the time of transfer," Dr. Madden continues, "it's so foreign from contemporary thinking about assisted reproduction, they're bound to become very upset. That's not the time to try to explain your reasons. So we have instituted an educational evening program near the beginning of the first treatment cycle that gives our patients an hour or two of information about what embryos do in the laboratory, and what are the implications of having a good-looking embryo, and the disadvantages of multiple births. This little minicourse helps them understand that no two people are alike and that just because your sister-in-law had four embryos transferred and delivered only one baby, doesn't mean that's what's best for you.

> *We have to help people think through the process. They need to understand the difficulties involved in a multiple gestation.*
>
> —JAMES MADDEN, M.D.

"So now our patients know from the beginning what to expect," he says. "They still have the final say, but now they are equipped to make a sound choice. Patient education has a huge role to play in the reduction of multiple gestations."

HOW OLD IS TOO OLD?

News headlines make getting pregnant sound so easy. The *Guinness Book of World Records 2001* lists the oldest moms as two 63-year-olds—one from California and one from Italy. A 60-year-old Japanese woman recently became her nation's oldest new mother when she gave birth to a healthy baby after undergoing in vitro fertilization in the United States. A Florida grandmother even delivered a baby son for her daughter. Although the majority of woman may not be waiting until their 60s to have children, pregnancies in older women are on the rise: The birthrate of first births for women in their 30s and 40s has surged in this country—quadrupling since 1970.[17] Celebrities add to the lure: Madonna bore a son at age 41, Jane Seymour gave birth to twins at age 44, and Susan Sarandon had a boy at age 45.

> *The birthrate of first births for women in their 30s and 40s has surged in this country—quadrupling since 1970.*

Sure, many women over 40 are healthy and fit. They look good, and they know they'll probably live long lives. But we shouldn't overlook the fact that advanced ART has certainly had a heavy hand in these births to older women.

No matter how fit a woman over 35 looks on the outside, inside her eggs are aging. This fact is relatively new news in the world of medical research, says Neil F. Goodman, M.D., a reproductive endocrinologist and clinical professor of medicine at the University of Miami School of Medicine. "It was only in the mid-1980s," he recalls, "that researchers discovered that eggs lose their fertility potential. While studying the success rates of IVF in certain age groups, Dr. Zev Rosenwaks in Virginia found that by age 35, there was a tremendous change in the success rate. And then the researchers began to examine why older women were having so much trouble conceiving and discovered that it was due to poor egg quality. It became apparent that

Been There, Done That: Coculture

You might hear about a futuristic-sounding idea called *embryo coculture* for IVF and wonder whether it will be available for you. Probably not. This is a process that looked good for a while but has already been assigned to the has-been dump in most cases. Using coculturing, IVF embryos are maintained in the laboratory for 3 or 4 days while being incubated with cells taken from the woman who will receive the embryos at transfer, rather than incubated in a synthetic medium. These cells may make some growth factor that is not fully understood at this time that could help stimulate embryonic growth or that could help remove toxins. (In the past, bovine cells from cows were successfully used, but the fear of disease transfer, especially after the outbreak of mad-cow disease, has ended that practice.)

As promising as coculturing seemed, it is a complex, time-consuming process that adds considerably to the expense of doing an IVF procedure. "To use the woman's own cells involves harvesting, biopsying, separating, cleaning, growing, and freezing," says Mark Perloe, M.D., medical director at Georgia Reproductive Specialists. All this contributes to the cost of IVF beyond any potential benefit in success rates. Given the improvement in the culture mediums available today that offer comparable success rates, there seems little benefit in using this procedure. It is rarely done."

even though a woman in her 40s might be having regular ovulatory cycles, the poor quality of her eggs might make it impossible for her to form normal embryos."

Dr. Gindoff notes, "This information was out there earlier, but it was buried in the literature. Only when older patients became more prevalent and conventional therapy failed did clinicians wake up to this phenomenon." The advances in reproductive science since the mid-1980s have not been able to change this biological fact.

But not to worry—ART to the rescue. Today's advances in IVF and donor egg transplant give many older women the gift of pregnancy, childbirth, and motherhood. Experts say, however, it may be a mistake to pin your hopes on a quick fix through IVF. The Centers for Disease Control has just published the 1999 IVF data gathered from 370 clinics in the United States, saying that the average pregnancy rate delivered per IVF cycle is about 30 percent.[18] On the one hand, these are impressive statistics for such a relatively new and complex procedure; on the other hand, they are not so comforting if you were counting on fail-proof conception. Any gambler knows the odds are against you with only a 30 percent chance of success. Many physicians working with infertile couples believe that too many women don't know the reality of these numbers.

That's why, as mentioned in the opening chapter, the ASRM launched a poster campaign in 2001 to warn women of the risk of waiting. The poster featured a baby's bottle shaped like an egg timer with a blunt accompanying message: "Advancing age decreases your ability to have children." The American Infertility Association has the same concerns and has been distributing pamphlets covering age-related fertility topics in doctors' offices across the country. These campaigns have sparked heated debates. Women who have been postponing pregnancy are furious at the implication that they are now somehow at fault for their infertility, while others are angry that no one mentioned this fact sooner.

> *Experts say it may be a mistake to pin your hopes on a quick fix through IVF.*

While this battle rages over when women should have children, other concerns are often voiced about "old-age" parenting. When ART is used to help younger couples achieve pregnancy, it is generally used to correct disease or a malfunctioning organ system. But when it is used in women over age 40, it is to reverse part of the normal aging process. This usage creates certain medical, pragmatic, and ethical concerns.

Medical Issues

An editorial in *The Lancet* reminded doctors that pregnancies in women over 40 are medically risky. It noted that these women have more hypertension during their pregnancies and more often hemorrhage after delivery. It also pointed out that they are more likely to need a cesarean section and suffer the consequences of major surgery. These maternal complications are all increased by multiple pregnancy—more common in ART pregnancies.[19] Another editorial in the *Journal of the American Medical Association* also discussed these risks, wondering whether there is an age beyond which a woman's organ systems are unable to adequately provide the nourishment required for a fetus's normal growth and development.[20]

> *When ART is used in women over age 40, it is to reverse part of the normal aging process. This usage creates certain medical, pragmatic, and ethical concerns.*

Practical Concerns

On the practical side, many wonder whether being able to have a baby in later life is as important as being able to raise that child. In her article, "Fertility and Folly," Jane Eisner voices the often unspoken, but obvious, concern when she says, "Trend-setting middle-age moms face the unenviable prospect of tussling with teenagers and pension arrangements at the same time. By having children later, they also diminish the chance that those children will have siblings, or cousins of a similar age, or be able to develop meaningful relationships with grandparents."[21] Still, others find no dilemma in older-age pregnancies and feel that an older parent is calmer, more understanding, and has more patience.

The Ethical Debate

A variety of ethical issues are also involved when using ART with older women. Most reproductive endocrinologists agree that there is no doubt that medical science has reached a point where it can establish a pregnancy in a 70-year-old woman. "Can we?" is no longer the question. The question many ask now is, "Should we?" Dr. Goodman has seen many wonderful advances in reproductive technology since he began working with infertile couples in 1974. These advances have allowed him to meet the goal he has dedicated his life's work to: helping infertile women conceive and carry to term. But now he finds himself facing the question, "Can the older woman carry the pregnancy to term without risking significant personal harm?"

> *Many wonder whether being able to have a baby in later life is as important as being able to raise that child.*

"Certainly we can put an embryo in her uterus and expect it to grow," he says, "but we don't know with any degree of certainty what the health hazards are for her compared to women in their 30s. We don't yet know how to do a prepregnancy evaluation of someone's cardiovascular system, for example, to determine the potential for heart failure due to the stress of pregnancy.

"The Hippocratic Oath cautions us to do no harm," continues Dr. Goodman, "and so at this point in time I believe it's unethical for a physician to help an older couple get pregnant when the risks to the mother cannot be clearly defined." Without any established standards to assess risk, many in the medical community have this same ethical concern about using ART for older women.

Looking more at the pragmatic side, others have questioned what will happen if late-life pregnancies become increasingly successful and the demand for donor eggs outstrips supply. Should young infertile women have first claim? Or, should older women with less time to wait be first in line? "And," adds Dr. Goodman, "who in our society will protect the rights of the child? Is it ethically sound to allow a 70-year-old couple to have a baby that will be orphaned in childhood?" None of these questions are easily answered and present the future challenge to using ART in older women.

PRESERVING FERTILITY

When a baby girl is born, her ovaries already contain a lifetime supply of eggs—about one million. No more will be made during her lifetime, and eventually (often around age 35) the eggs will begin to age and develop chromosomal abnormalities. The medical community is not able to change these facts at this time. Although research projects are in the works, no one has yet been able to force the ovary to produce new eggs or to stop the egg-aging process. But while the debate continues over how old is too old to have children, researchers continue to look for ways to preserve fertility and delay menopause. The three methods of fertility preservation grabbing the most attention are freezing eggs, freezing egg-containing ovarian tissue, and ovary implants.

Freezing Eggs

Fertility clinics around the world routinely freeze embryos created through IVF for later use, but it is rare to freeze eggs, which are more delicate and susceptible to damage from ice crystals during freezing. But on an experimental basis, some women are having their eggs frozen in the hopes that they will be able to use them at a later time.

Jeffrey Boldt, Ph.D., of the Assisted Fertility Services of Community Hospitals in Indianapolis, explains that "eggs are frozen by first treating them with chemicals called *cryoprotectants*. These chemicals help remove water from the egg so that damaging ice crystals do not form within the egg during freezing. The eggs are then placed into a special freezer and cooled slowly until placed into a liquid nitrogen tank for storage." At a later time, the eggs are slowly thawed and used for a subsequent attempt at an IVF conception.

This method has been used mainly for women with cancer who are facing sterilization from chemotherapy or radiation treatments. "Consider a 16-year-old girl," says Dr. Sable, "who develops Hodgkin's disease and has to undergo chemotherapy or radiation, which is likely to wipe out her population of usable eggs. Wouldn't it be nice to offer this girl 10 years later some option for regaining her fertility?" It is this hope that has fueled the research into freezing eggs that may someday give all women the opportunity to put off pregnancy and still have a biological child later in life.

About 20 babies worldwide have been conceived and born through this process, but it is certainly still considered experimental and under investigation.

Freezing Egg-Containing Ovarian Tissue

In 1999, a 30-year-old ballet dancer received the first ovarian tissue transplant and grabbed headlines when she then ovulated and had a menstrual period. At age 17, the young woman had had one of her ovaries removed when it developed a cyst. A year later the other ovary was removed. But in the hopes of preserving her fertility, before the second surgery her physicians removed and froze egg-containing slices from her ovary. Twelve years later, a physician in England who had been doing ovarian tissue transplant work on mice, thawed and stitched together 80 of the woman's ovarian slices and positioned them near the site of the original ovary. With the help of fertility hormones, the woman soon had a full menstrual cycle.

> *The promise of successfully using frozen ovarian tissue is an exciting advance over using frozen eggs alone.*

It is unclear how long the woman's apparent fertility will last, but the promise of successfully using frozen ovarian tissue is an exciting advance over using frozen eggs alone. Ovarian tissue slices are easier to obtain than individual eggs, and the immature eggs within are better able to survive the freezing and thawing process.[22]

Ovarian Implant

Kutluk Oktay, M.D., a reproductive endocrinologist at Cornell University, recently reported in the *Journal of the American Medical Association* the successful implant of ovarian tissue. Sections of ovaries were taken from two women and then implanted in their arms, where they continued to function. In both cases, the tissue produced visible welt-sized bumps in the forearm, just below the elbow. The tissue appeared to be functioning normally, and it has produced mature eggs and regulates the menstrual cycle. This offers hope that the women, both in their 30s, could become pregnant through IVF.

Dr. Oktay says the procedure could potentially benefit the estimated 40,000 to 50,000 U.S. women diagnosed each year with cancer during their reproductive years, who may require chemotherapy or radiation that can damage the ovaries. The tissue could be removed before treatment begins, then implanted in the arm after chemotherapy has finished and kept out of the way of radiation. "Thousands of others who take sterility-inducing drugs for ailments such as lupus and rheumatoid arthritis also could potentially benefit," says Dr. Oktay.[23]

Nonsurgical Options

Dr. Gindoff says that there are nonsurgical alternatives that should be offered to women before undergoing chemotherapy. "If women are treated with GnRH analogs that can shut down their ovaries and ovarian metabolism, the ovaries can remain dormant and protected for the most part from ill effects of the chemotherapy," he says. "This has shown promising results."

Cautious Optimism

These advances in preserving fertility offer much hope to tomorrow's women. But they are experimental and only in investigational stages right now, as Dr. Perloe adds a word of caution. "Do we harvest mature oocytes at age 25 to freeze for when a woman is 45? Or do we biopsy and freeze segments of ovary and either grow them in a lab or return them to the uterus at a later date? Do we know that we will end up with eggs that are not chromosomally damaged?

"We are at least 5 to 10 years away from the time when there is any reasonable chance that we'll know what we're doing when we do this," he says. "Right now these procedures are being performed, but the value of that tissue is questionable."

DECIDING THE FATE OF LEFTOVER EMBRYOS

The good news is that all 20 of your eggs are fertilized during an IVF procedure. The bad news is only four of these eggs will be transferred back into your uterus. So what will you do with the 16 leftover "babies"? This is a difficult decision facing many couples using today's ART procedures. As standard practice, most couples freeze the fertilized eggs for later use if the cycle fails or if they want more children at a later time. (More details about cryopreservation can be found in chapter 4.) But what should be done with the frozen embryos that are no longer wanted? There is no advanced technological answer to this basic question.

> *As standard practice, most couples freeze the fertilized eggs for later use if the cycle fails or if they want more children at a later time.*

Some couples find they cannot successfully carry transferred embryos and have no use for those they have fertilized and frozen. Some do have their child and do not want to go through another IVF procedure, leaving the fate of their frozen embryos in limbo. Other couples split up and now have the question of custody to work out. In these cases, there are generally four options: destroy the embryos, donate them to other infertile couples, donate them for research, or leave them in limbo—frozen in storage indefinitely.

Most couples sign a contract with the fertility clinic or hospital agreeing to a plan of action regarding unused embryos. But the law allows either partner to change his or her mind and amend the agreement, and therein lies the trouble. Although the legal status of embryos is unclear, many find themselves in the middle of court battles when couples disagree about their fate. For example, in 2001 the New Jersey Supreme Court rejected a man's attempts to have the leftover embryos from his prior marriage donated to another women against his ex-wife's wishes. The court expressed the opinion that no one should be forced to become a parent against his or her will. This ruling was only the fourth of its kind in the nation, and all four ended the same way. In Tennessee, New York, and Massachusetts, the parties wishing to avoid procreation all won their cases.[24] As these cases make their way to the Supreme Court, no doubt this issue of societal ethics will play a role in determining their outcome.

Spare Eggs for Research

Beyond the wishes of the couples involved with leftover embryos are the societal, moral, and ethical issues that affect the future of spare embryos. To many, destroying embryos as if they were no more than excess lab material is morally troubling, and this action sparks many heated debates—especially when the subject is using the embryos for stem cell research.

Stem cells are like the master cells of the body. They give rise to other cells the body needs for growth and maintenance. Those taken from a 5-day-old embryo have the power to divide indefinitely and create virtually all of the body's tissues. Scientists expect them to help generate tissue for treatment of disorders such as spinal cord injury, burns, juvenile diabetes, and stroke. They also are studying the cells to gain an understanding of human development and causes of birth defects and cancer.[25]

So what's the controversy? The sticky issue is the fact that human embryos are destroyed in the process of isolating stem cells. Some people object to this destruction of "life," while others argue that life does not begin until the nervous system appears 14 days after fertilization—long past the 5-day point of stem cell isolation. Even major religions differ on their beliefs about the onset of life for the embryo, fetus, or newborn, varying from conception, implantation, until even delivery. Some proponents remind protesters that the embryos used would be

> *Stem cells are like the master cells of the body. They give rise to other cells the body needs for growth and maintenance.*

those left over from IVF procedures, which would be destroyed anyway with no scientific gain. But opponents fear that eventually embryos will be created solely to be used for research purposes.

An interesting fact about stem cells that may calm the controversy is that they grow and divide indefinitely. This means that, in principle, the cells from just a single blastocyst could morph into virtually every kind of tissue, providing a potentially bottomless source. It is this aspect of stem cell production that prompted President George W. Bush to take a stand in August 2001 that he hoped would appease those against the destruction of human embryos as well as those seeking to use them to advance medical science. Bush announced that he would allow federal funding of research on embryonic stem cell lines already in existence (estimated to be approximately 60). But he would not allow federal funding for research that required the destruction of additional embryos that are routinely created and either frozen or discarded by fertility clinics.[26] Then eight months later, in April 2002, Bush called on Congress to render all types of human cloning illegal. This has set off ethical, legal and scientific debates in the field of embryology that we will be hearing much more about in the future.

Protecting Leftover Embryos

All this talk about what to do with leftover embryos often sidesteps the very real issue of ownership. When the politicians, courts, and doctors are debating whether the fertilized eggs should be destroyed, donated to infertile couples, or used for research, it is rare to hear from the couples who own those eggs. In fact, it is not unheard of for the fate of embryos to be decided without even asking for the consent of the "parents."

Thanks in large part to the efforts of Melanie Blum, a California attorney specializing in reproductive law, California is the only state in the country to pass legislation making it a felony to implant human embryos or eggs or utilize them for research purposes without the donor's written consent. This law was passed after Blum represented couples in the landmark case against the University of California, Irvine, and its now-defunct Center for Reproductive Health, alleging that patients' eggs and embryos were stolen and sold to other patients. Yes, this happens, and in your state it may not be against the law. "I'm representing a woman right now," says Blum, "who donated eggs for one other woman to use. The doctor split the eggs between two women because he felt the shortage of eggs and embryos gave him the right to use the eggs in whatever way he wanted."

Blum feels that couples need to know that this sort of behavior happens and choose their doctors carefully. "Eggs are taken out of the body at a time when the women are under a general anesthetic," she explains. "They have no way of counting these microscopic eggs. They have to completely trust their physician. The extra embryos are then frozen and stored, but they still belong to the couple. Only the patient can consent to removing them." But this doesn't always happen. "In some cases," continues Blum, "the clinics destroy or distribute stored embryos without notifying the owners."

California is the only state in the country to pass legislation making it a felony to implant human embryos or eggs or utilize them for research purposes without the donor's written consent.

Blum has some words of advice if you have leftover embryos in storage: "Make sure you have your storage fees paid up," she says. "And constantly check on the status of your embryos. Every time you pay your bill, request an update of the tank inventory. You want to make sure that nothing has changed and the numbers of your embryos are consistent from year to year. Also, make sure your clinic requires a notarized signature to make any changes to the embryo status. I'm representing a client right now whose wife went to the clinic during the time of their divorce proceedings and forged the husband's signature trying to get the embryos donated to another couple. I can go on and on about these kinds of cases involving embryos."

The point is, in most cases, there are no laws yet to protect you and your embryos. "In the future, I would like to see federal legislation that incorporates these issues of family law, reproductive law, and contract law," says Blum. "We need to recognize that we have new ways of creating families, and we need to uniformly regulate the protection of eggs and embryos. No couple should ever be surprised to find out that someone else has received their embryo and has given birth to their child."

SERIOUS INSURANCE CONCERNS

No one debates that infertility testing and treatment is expensive. One IVF cycle alone can run up a total cost of $20,000. The question that stirs controversy is, "Who should pay for it?" Many health insurers and employers oppose insurance coverage, claiming that infertility is not a disease. Having children, they feel, is a lifestyle choice that they should not have to pay for (although they cover other diseases associated with lifestyle choices such as lung disease due to cigarette smoking). Some will cover infertility caused by a specific medical condition (e.g., endometriosis) but will not cover situations such as unexplained infertility (feeling it is probably the luck of the genetic draw, like the color of one's skin or length of the nose) or infertility caused by age (feeling that if you wait too long it's your own fault, which forfeits your right to an insurance claim). Others say the cost of infertility coverage is just too high and will boost the rates of all subscribers. In addition, many feel that the success rate per treatment is too low to justify the cost of coverage.

Many health insurers and employers oppose insurance coverage, claiming that infertility is not a disease.

On the other side of the argument are infertile couples and their doctors who believe that infertility is a medical condition and should be treated as such. Kate Doyle, the director of government affairs for RESOLVE, says, "Infertility is a physical problem that can be corrected by medical treatments. Everyone should have the right and the ability to have a family, but some need assistance to have that family."[27]

Advocates for insurance coverage point to states that have mandatory infertility coverage and do not suffer exorbitant rates. They also protest the unfairness of insurance companies that cover the cost of Viagra (the drug used to treat erectile dysfunction in men) but not infertility medical treatment. As explained more fully in the section "Dealing with the Problems of Higher-Order Multiples," it's also known that the degree of insurance coverage affects the likelihood of multiple births (costing the insurance companies far more than infertility coverage would have cost) because couples with no or limited insurance coverage try to increase their chances of success by stimulating more eggs or transferring more embryos.

Get the Facts About Insurance

As the debate continues, you must become your own insurance advocate to make sure that if you are entitled to coverage, you get it. The degree of services covered by health insurance companies depends on where you live and the type of insurance plan you have. Only 14 states mandate insurance coverage for infertility at this time: Arkansas, California, Connecticut, Hawaii, Illinois, Maryland, Massachusetts, Montana, New Jersey, New York, Ohio, Rhode Island, Texas, and West Virginia.

> *You must become your own insurance advocate to make sure that if you are entitled to coverage, you get it.*

That mandate, however, does not mean that you are automatically covered. What exactly the mandate covers varies from state to state, and in some states there's an interesting twist: The mandates require insurance carriers to offer infertility coverage but does not require employers to take that option and provide infertility coverage. You'll see that some mandates apply only to employers with more than 50 employees. Some apply to insurance carriers but not HMOs. Others require coverage for diagnosis but not treatment. Some exclude IVF and others cover only IVF. Some offer coverage for "diagnosis and treatment of

Resource Referral

For more information about state laws and infertility insurance coverage, contact your state insurance commissioner, or visit the ASRM's Web site and click on "State Infertility Insurance Laws" at www.asrm.org/patients/insur.html.

correctable medical conditions" and then exclude IVF as a corrective treatment. Some have age limitations.

If you are one of the lucky ones who has insurance coverage for infertility testing and diagnosis, don't assume too much about that coverage. Let's say you've been told that if your policy doesn't specifically state that infertility is excluded from coverage, then you're covered. In theory this may be true, but there are all sorts of ways the carrier can still limit what it will pay. You have to find out exactly what is mandated in your state and what is covered in your insurance contract. Ask to see your insurance contract (which may be different from the policy that is sent to you in the mail). Federal law gives you a right to see this contract within 30 days of a request.

Christina Schlank, who wrote the book, *Medicine and Money*, says you must have answers to certain questions before you begin medical care for infertility. She recommends that you check your insurance policy and talk to your insurance representative or human resource person to find the answers to these questions:

- Is there a preexisting condition limitation? (If you buy or become covered by an employer's policy after your infertility is diagnosed, a preexisting condition clause could make you ineligible for coverage, even though that policy offers full infertility coverage.)

- What is the deductible copayment for infertility treatments and medications?

- Is there an annual out-of-pocket cost?

- Does the policy dictate the types of treatments covered or the order in which the procedures are performed?

- Do you need separate referrals for each medical doctor you see? (You may go to one doctor for diagnosis and another for treatment or even another for a different form of treatment.)

- What is the maximum payout allowed for infertility treatments?

Be especially cautious about information you receive from an insurance representative over the telephone. You have no way of knowing

---

Medical Hero or Outlaw?

In some cases, doctors have found ways around insurance limitations on infertility procedures. They have been known to perform an IUI or IVF that is not covered by a couple's policy and then bill the insurance company for a fertility "treatment" like surgery that is covered. This practice was not uncommon across the country, but after the conviction of Dr. Niels Lauersen in 2001 on insurance fraud charges, it may suddenly be hard to find a doctor willing to take such risks again.

Dr. Lauersen was a renowned infertility specialist from New York City whose patients included such high-profile names as Celine Dion and Liv Ullmann. Prosecutors said he helped women get pregnant by providing fertility treatments not covered by insurance. Then he submitted bills for reimbursement for various covered treatments. His defense attorney argued for leniency saying that the doctor had an honorable purpose—to make it affordable for women with fertility problems to have a child. Dr. Lauersen was sentenced to seven years in prison and ordered to pay $3.2 million in restitution and $17,000 in fines.[28]

whether that person has any idea what he or she is talking about. You may be told that you are covered for three IUIs, so you arrange for the procedure, and then find out your policy does not cover IUI at all. "But that's what I was told on the phone" means nothing at that point. Schlank advises, "It's best to call, get the name of the person you're talking to, and ask your questions; then write down the information you receive, send it in a letter to the insurance company and ask them to verify that the information is correct and give you preauthorization."

Infertility and Disability

Adding to the debate over whether infertility is a disease, recent cases have asked the courts to define infertility as a disability. Schlank explains: "The Americans with Disabilities Act (ADA) defines an individual with a disability as a person who has a physical or mental impairment that substantially limits one or more major life activities." Recently the courts have been using this definition to rule in favor of couples who sue their employers and insurance companies for offering policies that discriminate against gender and disability by denying infertility coverage. There has been no sweeping proclamation that all infertility cases are covered under this act, but on a case-by-case basis, some couples are gaining coverage through this door. Of course, under the ADA laws, there is a safe-harbor clause for employers to avoid covering these treatments if they can prove that such coverage would cause a financial hardship. But it's one avenue to consider if your employer refuses to offer the option of infertility coverage.

Schlank reminds us that insurance is a consumer-driven business. "Insurance companies need customers to make a profit," she says, "and they respond to political and consumer pressure. It may be a battle, but if the pressure for coverage continues, they may eventually have to give in."

The truth of this statement is evident in New Jersey—the 14th state to mandate insurance coverage for infertility treatment. During a 6-year battle, 2,500 people waged an almost daily e-mail and letter

> **Behind the Scenes**
>
> A lot of research is going on in laboratories all over the country that in unheralded but significant ways is contributing to the knowledge needed to understand infertility fully. For example, Keith Blackwell, M.D., Ph.D., an investigator at the Center for Blood Research at Harvard Medical School, is examining the problem of oocyte (unfertilized egg) competence and survival. His recent work found a molecule that is essential for oocyte survival, shedding light on how/why the vast numbers of oocytes die in a kind of culling process of "defective" oocytes. This is the kind of knowledge that improves the store of reproductive information needed to help infertile couples in the future.

campaign to state legislators. They were lucky to find a few legislators who had their own infertility problems and who willingly supported the bill, creating a perfect mix of consumer and political pressure.

THE CLONING DEBATE

The news of asexual animal cloning around the world holds potentially relevant information for infertile couples. When scientists cloned CC the cat in 2002, the team painstakingly fused 188 skin cells with cat eggs whose own DNA had been removed, creating 82 cloned embryos that were transferred to the wombs of seven cats. One pregnancy resulted but ended in miscarriage. In a second effort, the team transferred five cloned embryos to a surrogate mother cat—three of them made from ovarian tissue cells, rather than skin cells, taken from an adult cat. This time the effort was successful, and CC was born.[29]

CC is the sixth kind of mammal to be created asexually from a single adult cell; sheep, mice, cattle, goats, and pigs have already passed the test. The next logical step in the pursuit of science is human cloning, which is no longer the stuff of science fiction.

In November 2001, the research company, Advanced Cell Technology in Worcester, Massachusetts, claimed to have cloned a human being. The researchers took a woman's donated egg cell and sucked out the nucleus with its genetic core. Then they took a separate cumulus cell, which nurtures a developing egg, and injected it whole (with its own genetic material) into the egg cells. The cloned cumulus cell grew into a primitive sex-cell embryo. It is too early to say whether such an embryo could be transferred into a woman's womb and grow into a human child.[30]

That possibility, say the researchers, is not the point of this spectacular discovery. Rather than pursue human reproductive cloning (which is banned in several states and awaiting federal ban from Congress), the goal of these experiments is to explore therapeutic cloning.

Therapeutic cloning is performed to obtain stem cells from the cloned embryo that are identical to the cell donor. When this happens, the stem cells can be manipulated to create compatible replacement tissue. Advocates are excited about the possibility of using this procedure to find a cure for diseases such as heart disease, diabetes, Alzheimer's, Parkinson's, and other degenerative diseases, as well as reversal of spinal cord injuries.

> *R*ather than pursue human reproductive cloning (which is banned in several states and awaiting federal ban from Congress), the goal of these experiments is to explore therapeutic cloning.

A first step in this direction was taken again by Advanced Cell Technology, when in January 2002, it announced a successful attempt at using cloning technology to grow genetically matched organs for transplantation. The scientists used cells derived from cloned cow embryos to grow kidney-like organs that function and are not rejected when implanted into adult cows. If the approach could be used to make human kidneys from cloned human embryos, it could dramatically reduce the need for donor kidneys and transplants in the future.[31]

So What's the Holdup?

There are many exciting and bold ideas and theories among the thousands of medical researchers studying infertility. But these ideas are slow to grow into successful practice. Because many of the experiments involve the swapping of cell parts—a process that uses some of the same steps involved in cloning—the Federal Drug Administration has stepped in, warning researchers that they must submit to the arduous process of biological drug approval before continuing to experiment with human cells.[32]

These findings might influence the outcome of the upcoming Senate vote on the Human Cloning Prohibition Act, which would ban the kind of research that led to this discovery. Many people consider research on human embryo clones unethical and have called for a federal ban on the procedure. But others believe that such objections might be outweighed if the research were shown to be the most promising means of growing compatible replacement tissues.

Similar to the way researchers, physicians, lawyers, politicians, and society as a whole debated the use of in vitro fertilization on moral and ethical grounds back in 1978 when Louise Brown became the first "test-tube" baby, the human cloning debate promises to be an equally sensitive and divisive issue.

THE HOPE OF TODAY

Undoubtedly, the treatment of infertility will change in future years and generations. There will most likely be a time, when despite infertility, a couple will be able to conceive, carry, and deliver a healthy baby without the physical risks caused by fertility drugs, without the emotional devastation of repeated failed cycles, and without the financial burden of no or limited insurance coverage.

But that day is in the future. For now, the available methods of infertility treatment are all you have. Although not perfect, they are far more than what was available just a generation ago. And they are enough to give you hope that despite infertility, you can give birth to a child of your own.

Appendix: Resources

SUPPORT AND INFORMATIONAL ORGANIZATIONS

Adoption, Donors, and Surrogacy Families 2000
200 Newport Center Drive,
    Suite 203
Newport Beach, CA 92660
Phone: (800) 990-BABY
E-mail: info@families2000.com
Web site: www.families2000.com

Adoptive Families of America
3333 Highway 100 North
Minneapolis, MN 55422
Phone: (800) 372-3300

American Academy of Medical Acupuncture
4929 Wilshire Boulevard,
    Suite 428
Los Angeles, CA 90010
Phone: (323) 937-5514
Web site: www.medical
    acupuncture.org

American Association of Clinical Endocrinologists
1000 Riverside Avenue, Suite 205
Jacksonville, FL 32204
Phone: (904) 353-7878
Fax: (904) 353-8185
Web site: www.aace.com

American Association of Naturopathic Physicians
8201 Greensboro Drive, Suite 300
McLean, VA 22102
Phone: (877) 969-2267 or
    (703) 610-9037
Web site: www.naturopathic.org

American Society for Reproductive Medicine
1209 Montgomery Highway
Birmingham, AL 35216
Phone: (205) 978-5000
Web site: www.asrm.org

American Society of Andrology
2950 Buskirk Avenue, Suite 170
Walnut Creek, CA 94596
Phone: (925) 472-5910
Fax: (925) 472-5901
E-mail: asa@hp-assoc.com
Web site: www.andrologysociety
  .com

**InterNational Council on
Infertility Information
Dissemination (INCIID)**
P.O. Box 91363
Tucson, AZ 85752
Phone: (520) 554-9548
Web site: www.inciid.org

**The National Adoption
Information Clearinghouse**
5540 Nicholson Lane, Suite 300
Rockville, MD 20852
Phone: (301) 231-6512

**National Center for
Homeopathy (NCH)**
801 N. Fairfax Street, Suite 306
Alexandria, Virginia 22314
Phone: (877) 624-0613 or
  (703) 548-7790
Web site: www.homeopathic.org.

**National Certification
Commission for Acupuncture
and Oriental Medicine**
11 Canal Center Plaza, Suite 300
Alexandria, VA 22314
Phone: (703) 548-9004
E-mail: info@nccaom.org
Web site: www.nccaom.org

**National Women's Health
Information Center**
8550 Arlington Blvd., Suite 300
Fairfax, VA 22031
Phone: (800) 994-9662
Web site: www.4woman.gov

**Polycystic Ovarian Syndrome
Association, Inc.**
P.O. Box 80517
Portland, OR 97280
Phone: (877) 775-7267
E-mail: info@pcosupport.org
Web site: www.pcosupport.org

**RESOLVE (also known as the
National Infertility Association)**
1310 Broadway
Somerville, MA 02144
Phone: (888) 623-0744
Web site: www.resolve.org

Surrogate Alternatives, Inc.
13460 Huntington Street
Fontana, CA 92336
Phone: (909) 899-9611
E-mail: surrogacy4U@aol.com
Web site: www.surrogate
  alternatives.net

INFORMATIVE WEB SITES

The American Infertility Association
www.americaninfertility.org

The American Journal of Bioethics Online
www.bioethics.net

CDC Reproductive Health Information Source
www.cdc.gov/nccdphp/drh
   /art98/index.htm

The Center for Advanced Reproductive Services
www.fertilitycenter-uconn.org
   /education.htm

Child of My Dreams
www.childofmydreams.com

Egg Donation, Inc.
www.eggdonor.com

Fertile Thoughts
www.fertilethoughts.net

The Institute for Reproductive Medicine and Science of Saint Barnabas
www.sbivf.com

Internet Health Resources
www.ihr.com

IVF.com
www.ivf.com

Obgyn.net
www.obgyn.net

Reproductive Endocrinology & Infertility
www.med.nyu.edu/ObGyn
   /DivEndo.html

Shared Journey
www.sharedjourney.com

The Visible Embryo
www.visembryo.com

FURTHER READING

The Couple's Guide to Fertility by Gary S. Berger, Marc Goldstein, and Mark L. Fuerst (New York: Broadway Books, 2001).

Dr. Richard Marrs' Fertility Book by Richard Marrs (New York: Dell Books, 1998).

The Fertility Sourcebook by M. Sara Rosenthal (Los Angeles: Lowell House, 1998).

The Infertility Survival Guide by Judith C. Daniluk (Oakland, CA: New Harbinger, 2001).

Natural Fertility by Francesca Naish (Bowral, Australia: Milner, 2000).

Rewinding Your Biological Clock: Motherhood Late in Life: Options, Issues, and Emotions by Richard J. Paulson and Judith Sachs (New York: Freeman, 2000).

6 Steps to Increased Fertility by Robert Barbieri, Alice Domar, and Kevin Loughlin (New York: Simon & Schuster 2000).

Notes

Chapter 1

1. MayoClinic.com, "Male Infertility: Causes and Remedies," *Reproductive Health*, www.mayoclinic.com/home?id=HO00103, 2000.

2. J. Jarrett and D. Rausch, *The Fertility Guide* (Santa Fe, NM: Health Press, 1998).

3. C.L. Mithers, "Why Can't I Have Another Baby?" *Ladies' Home Journal* 118 (August 2001): 68.

4. S. Silber, *How to Get Pregnant with the New Technology* (New York: Warner, 1991): 52.

5. Ibid. 53.

6. H. MacGregor, "Women Assaulted by a Stork Reality: Doctor-Sponsored Poster Campaign Warns of Difficulty Conceiving as Women Grow Older," *Los Angeles Times*, August 31, 2001, part 5, 1.

7. S. Jordan, "Women Face Countdown to Infertility," *Observer News*, August 12, 2001, 20.

8. American Society for Reproductive Medicine, "Patient's Fact Sheet: Infertility," www.asrm.org/Patients/FactSheets/Infertility-Fact.pdf, 1997.

9. Georgia Reproductive Specialists, "Fast Facts on Infertility" (handout); and D.M. de Kretser, "Male Infertility," *The Lancet* 349 (March 15, 1997): 787.

10. MacGregor, "Women Assaulted by a Stork Reality."

11. J. Aiman, "A History of Human Fertility," in *Infertility: Diagnosis and Management*, ed. J. Aiman (New York: Springer, 1984).

12. M. Larkin, "Male Reproductive Health: A Hotbed of Research," *The Lancet* 352 (August 15, 1998): 552.

13. American Society for Reproductive Medicine, "Patient's Fact Sheet: Infertility."

14. D.L. Healy, A. Trounson, and A. Andersen, "Female Infertility: Causes and Treatment," *The Lancet* 343 (June 18, 1994): 1539.

15. Ibid.

16. American Academy of Family Physicians, "Polycystic Ovary Syndrome," *American Family Physician* 62 (September 1, 2000): 1090.

17. Jarrett and Rausch, *The Fertility Guide*.

18. M.S. Rosenthal, *The Fertility Sourcebook* (Los Angeles: Lowell House, 1998).

19. World Health Organization, "The Influence of Varicocele on Parameters of Fertility in a Large Group of Men Presenting to Infertility Clinics," *Fertility Sterility* 57 (1992): 1289.

20. L. Nachtigall, P. Boepple, F. Pralong, and W. Crowley, "Adult-Onset Idiopathic Hypogonadotropic Hypogonadism: A Treatable Form of Male Infertility," *New England Journal of Medicine* 336 (February 6, 1997): 410.

21. Mithers, "Why Can't I Have Another Baby?"

22. R. Munkelwitz and B. Gilbert, "Are Boxer Shorts Really Better? A Critical Analysis of the Role of Underwear Type in Male Subfertility," *Journal of Urology* 160 (October 1998): 1329–1333.

23. "Fecundity of Males Is Found to Decline After the Age of 24." *Wall Street Journal*, August 9, 2000, B7a.

24. Silber, *How to Get Pregnant with the New Technology*.

25. D. Guzick, "When Infertility Can't Be Explained," *Contemporary OB/GYN* 45 (September 2000): 102.

Chapter 2

1. D.N. Clapp, "Fact Sheet 16: Selecting an Infertility Physician," RESOLVE, www.resolve.org/special.htm, June 2000.

2. M. Perloe and L. Christie, *Miracle Babies* (New York: Rawson, 1986).

3. D.N. Clapp, "Fact Sheet 16: Selecting an Infertility Physician," RESOLVE, www.resolve.org/special.htm, June 2000. Reprinted with permission.

4. M. Goldstein and P. Schlegel, "The Fertility Evaluation," Center for Male Reproductive Medicine and Microsurgery, www.maleinfertility.org, March 5, 2001.

5. NewsRx, "Bacteria in Semen Linked to Reduced Fertility," *Impotence & Male Health Weekly Plus*, NewsRx.com, October 26, 1998.

6. American Society for Reproductive Medicine, "Fact Sheet: Diagnostic Testing for Male Factor Infertility," www.asrm.org/Patients/FactSheets/Testing_Male-Fact.pdf, February 1997.

7. P. Landesman, "Missing Children," *Men's Health* 13 (September 1998): 175.

8. American Society for Reproductive Medicine, "Fact Sheet: Diagnostic Testing for Male Factor Infertility."

9. Ibid.

10. NewsRx, "Link Made to Male Infertility," *Cancer Weekly*, NewsRx.com, October 17, 2000.

11. K. Frey, M. Stenchever, and M. Warren, "Helping the Infertile Couple," *Patient Care* 23 (May 30, 1989): 22.

12. Ibid.

13. Penton Media, Inc., "A Test Solution," *Industry Week* 245 (June 3, 1996): 15.

14. M. Applebaum, "Sonohysterography: A Safer Alternative to Hysterography," www.inciid.org/hsg-sono.html, 1998.

15. Clinical Reference Systems, "Diagnostic Laparoscopy for Infertility," *Annual 2000* (2000): 490.

16. K. Johnson, "Finding Pathology in 'Normal' Infertility Patients," *OB GYN News* 35 (March 1, 2000): 18.

Chapter 3

1. L. Goldstein, "Can Cough Syrup Help You Get Pregnant?" *Prevention* 52 (April 2000): 194.

2. F. Reiss, *The Infertility Diet: Get Pregnant and Prevent Miscarriage* (Newton, MA: Peanut Butter and Jelly Press, 1999).

3. G. Berger, *The Couple's Guide to Fertility* (New York: Doubleday, 1989).

4. D.L. Healy, A. Trounson, and A. Andersen, "Female Infertility: Causes and Treatment," *The Lancet* 343 (June 18, 1994): 1539.

5. F. Naish, *Natural Fertility* (Bowral, Australia: Milner, 2000).

6. C. Henderson, "Some of Smoking's Harmful Effects Reserved Specifically for Women," *Women's Health Weekly* (December 7, 2000): 13.

7. D. Hollander, "Conception May Take a Long Time Among Women Who Smoke," *Family Planning Perspectives* 28 (July–August 1996): 181.

8. W. Conkling, *Getting Pregnant Naturally* (New York: Avon, 1999).

9. R. Smoak, "Smoking and Impotence: Hitting Below the Belt," *American Medical News* (November 2, 1998): 17.

10. "Caffeine Intake and Delayed Conception," *Nutrition Research Newsletter* 16 (May 1997): 58.

11. Conkling, *Getting Pregnant Naturally*, 130.

12. M. Perloe and L. Christie, *Miracle Babies* (New York: Rawson, 1986).

13. Conkling, *Getting Pregnant Naturally*, 131.

14. M. Napoli, "Calcium Channel Blockers: Causes Male Infertility," *HealthFacts* (November 1999).
15. Berger, *The Couple's Guide to Fertility*.
16. American Society for Reproductive Medicine, "Patient's Fact Sheet: Exercise, Weight, and Fertility," www.asrm.org/Patients/FactSheets/Exercise-Fact.pdf, 1996.
17. NewsRX, "Being Underweight or Overweight Reduces Probability of Pregnancy," *Women's Health Weekly* (December 21, 2000): 20.
18. R. Winston, *What We Know About Infertility* (New York: Free Press 1986).
19. P. Landesman, "Missing Children," *Men's Health* 13 (September 1998): 174.
20. "Is Driving a Risk Factor for Male Infertility?" *Contemporary Urology* 12 (November 2000): 88.
21. Berger, *The Couple's Guide to Fertility*.
22. K. Thorson, "Acupuncture: Is It for You?" *Fibromyalgia Network Newsletter* (January 2000): 9.
23. D. Ni, "Chinese Medicine and Reproductive Medicine," lecture presented to the Pacific Coast Reproductive Society, Santa Monica, CA, April 15, 1999.
24. American Academy of Medical Acupuncture, "Frequently Asked Questions About Medical Acupuncture," www.medicalacupuncture.org/acu_info/faqs.html.
25. J. Horstman, "Acupuncture," *Arthritis Today* (May–June 2000): 78.
26. National Center for Homeopathy, "Introduction to Homeopathy," www.homeopathic.org.
27. T. Monmaney and S. Roan, "Hope or Hype?" www.latimes.com, August 30, 1998.
28. Ni, "Chinese Medicine and Reproductive Medicine."
29. J. Brody, "Herbal Remedies Tied to Pregnancy Risks," *New York Times*, March 9, 1999, 7.
30. InterNational Council on Infertility Information Dissemination, "Alternative Therapies Disclaimer," www.inciid.org/forums/alternatives/index.html.

Chapter 4

1. American Society for Reproductive Medicine, "Patient's Fact Sheet: Infertility" www.asrm.org/Patients/FactSheets/Infertility-Fact.pdf, 1997.
2. American Society for Reproductive Medicine, "Frequently Asked Questions About Infertility," www.asrm.com/patients/faqs.html, 2001.

3. M.S. Rosenthal, *The Fertility Sourcebook* (Los Angeles: Lowell House, 1998).

4. Micromedex, "Advice for the Patient: Drug Information in Lay Language; Annual 2001," *USP DI*, Vol. II (2001): 642.

5. "Fertility Drugs: Make an Educated Choice," Fertility Challenges and Therapies, www.mayoclinic.com/home, January 29, 2001.

6. D. Keefe, "Use of Crinone Demonstrates Excellent Pregnancy Rates," *American Family Physician* 61 (April 15, 2000): 2472.

7. American Society for Reproductive Medicine, "Fact Sheet: Risks of In Vitro Fertilization," www.asrm.com/patients/invitro/risks, December 1996.

8. "Fertility Drugs."

9. Ibid.

10. "Treating Infertility: ARTs Offer Help," Fertility Challenges and Therapies, www.mayoclinic.com/home, January 9, 2001.

11. D.L. Healy, A. Trounson, and A. Andersen, "Female Infertility: Causes and Treatment," *The Lancet* 343 (June 18, 1994): 1539.

12. Rosenthal, *The Fertility Sourcebook*.

13. "Infertility: Male: Diseases and Conditions A–Z," www.mayoclinic.com/home?id=5.1.1.9.6#Treatment, August 8, 2001.

14. M. Goldstein, P. Schlegel, and P. Shihua, "The Fertility Evaluation." Center for Male Reproductive Medicine and Microsurgery, www.male infertility.org, March 5, 2001.

15. S. Silber, *How to Get Pregnant with the New Technology* (New York: Warner, 1991).

16. Ibid.

17. American Society for Reproductive Medicine, "Frequently Asked Questions About Infertility."

18. National Institutes of Health, "NICHD Network Identifies Most Effective of a Series of Infertility Treatments," *NIH News Alert*, www.nichd.nih.gov/new/releases/FERTR199.htm, January 21, 1999.

19. "Infertility: Male: Diseases and Conditions A–Z."

20. WGBH Educational Foundation, "18 Ways to Make a Baby," NOVA #2811, www.pbs.org/wgbh/nova/transcripts/2811baby.html, October 9, 2001.

21. American Society for Reproductive Medicine, "Fact Sheet: In Vitro Fertilization (IVF)," www.asrm.com/patients/factsheets/invitro.html, 2001.

22. WGBH Educational Foundation, "18 Ways to Make a Baby."

23. American Society for Reproductive Medicine, "Fact Sheet: Intracytoplasmic Sperm Injection," www.asrm.org/patients/factsheets/icsi-fact.pdf, August 2001.

24. M. Napoli, "IVF Without Simulation Drugs Almost as Successful," *Health Facts* (March 2001).

25. Goldstein et al., "The Fertility Evaluation."

26. A. Warren, "Father's Day Miracles," *Family Circle* 110 (June 24, 1997): 92.

27. G. Berger, *The Couple's Guide to Fertility* (New York: Doubleday, 1989).

28. American Society for Reproductive Medicine, "Fact Sheet: Intracytoplasmic Sperm Injection."

29. D. Goenka, "7th ISAR Pre-Congress Andrology Workshop," *Newsletter International Society of Andrology*, www.andrology.org/directory/fertility/goenka.html, 2001.

30. K. Hsu, "Risk Seen of Passing Male Infertility Along in Reproductive Bid," *Boston Globe*, July 1, 1999, A1.

31. WGBH Educational Foundation, "18 Ways to Make a Baby."

32. The Valley Hospital, "Center for In Vitro Fertilization and Reproductive Endocrinology Make Dreams of Parenthood a Reality," *Valley Reports* (Fall 2001): 8.

33. "Infertility: Male: Diseases and Conditions A–Z."

34. C. Kurdas, "Reproductive Medicine: New Findings," *Contemporary Ob/Gyn* (November 1999): 128.

35. C. Henderson, "Two Methods of Implanting Embryos Yield Similar Success Rates," *Women's Health Weekly* (November 23, 2000): 9.

36. Ibid.

37. American Society for Reproductive Medicine, "Fact Sheet: Intracytoplasmic Sperm Injection."

38. C. Henderson, "Researchers Explore Ways to Preserve Female Fertility," *Women's Health Weekly* (December 7, 2000): 12.

39. K. Uhlenhuth, "Just How Are Embryos Stored and for How Long?" *Kansas City Star*, August 28, 2001, E1.

Chapter 5

1. M. Quigley, "The New Frontier of Reproductive Age," *Journal of the American Medical Association* 268 (September 9, 1992): 1320.

2. R. Laliberte, "To Make a Baby, Click Here," *Redbook* (September 1999): 122.

3. S. Lerner, "Egg Hunt," *Village Voice* (August 17, 1999): 26.

4. C. Goldberg, "On Web, Models Auction Their Eggers to Bidders for Beautiful Children," *New York Times*, October 23, 1999, A11.

5. "Couple Offers $100,000 in Ad Seeking Woman to Donate Eggs." *Los Angeles Times*, February 9, 2000, A20.

6. Surrogate Mothers, Inc., "General Information," www.surrogatemothers
.com/info.htm, 2001.

7. Ibid.

8. K.S. Stolley, "Statistics on Adoption in the United States," *The Future of Children: Adoption* 3 (1993): 26–42.

9. V. Flango and C. Flango, *The Flow of Adoption Information from the States* (Williamsburg, VA: National Center for State Courts, 1994).

10. M. Tucker, "Foreign Children Present Unique Infectious Disease Issues," *Family Practice News* 31 (January 15, 2001): 6.

11. M. Cain, *The Childless Revolution* (Cambridge, MA: Perseus, 2001).

Chapter 6

1. L. Glover, P.D. Abel, and K. Gannon, "Male Subfertility: Is Pregnancy the Only Issue?" *British Medical Journal* 316 (May 9, 1998): 1405.

2. P. Landesman, "Missing Children," *Men's Health* 13 (September 1998): 174.

3. Ibid.

4. J. Daniluk, *The Infertility Survival Guide* (Oakland, CA: New Harbinger, 2001).

5. L. Peterson, "Why Join a Support Group?" www.resolve.org/supgroups
.html.

6. A. Katz, ed., H. Hedrich, and C.E. Koop, *Self-Help: Concepts and Applications* (Philadelphia: Charles, 1992).

7. R. Barbieri, A. Domar, and K. Loughlin, *6 Steps to Increased Fertility* (New York: Simon & Schuster 2000).

8. American Society for Reproductive Medicine, "Fact Sheet: Stress and Infertility," www.asrm.org/Patients/FactSheets/Stress-Fact.pdf, September 1996.

9. J. Lasater, "When You Want to Have a Baby . . . but Can't," *Yoga Journal* (November 2001): 96.

10. Association for Applied Psychophyisiology and Biofeedback, "What Is Biofeedback?" www.aapb.org/public/articles/details.cfm?id=4, 2001.

11. Touch Research Institute, "Aromatherapy's Effect on Moods and Minds," *International Journal of Neuroscience* 96 (1998): 217–224.

12. M. Cameron and T. DiGeronimo, *Mother Nature's Guide to Vibrant Beauty and Health* (Paramus, NJ: Prentice Hall, 1997).

13. E. Nagourney, "Vital Signs: Fertility." *New York Times*, October 2, 2001, F6.

14. American Yoga Association, "General Yoga Information," www.american
yogaassociation.org.

15. Lasater, "When You Want to Have a Baby . . . but Can't."

16. Barbieri et al., *6 Steps to Increased Fertility*.

17. National Institutes of Mental Health, "If You're over 65 and Feeling Depressed," NIH publication no. 95-4033, www.nimh.nih.gov/publicat /over65.cfm, 1995.

Chapter 7

1. E. McClam, "CDC: Fertility Procedures on Rise," *AOL Health News*, AOL.com, February 7, 2002.

2. Ibid.

3. Ibid.

4. M.S. Rosenthal, *The Fertility Sourcebook* (Los Angeles: Lowell, 1998).

5. WGBH Educational Foundation, "18 Ways to Make a Baby," NOVA #2811, www.pbs.org/wgbh/nova/transcripts/2811baby.html, October 9, 2001.

6. American Society for Reproductive Medicine, "Fact Sheet: Preimplantation Genetic Diagnosis," www.asrm.org/Patients/FactSheets/PGD-Fact .pdf, 1998.

7. Saint Barnabas Health Care Systems, "New Data on Genetic Testing of Embryos Before Transplantation Shows Reduction in Miscarriages and Improved Chance of Normal Pregnancy," www.sbhcs.com/news /embryos.html.

8. J. B. Younger, "ASRM Position on Gender Selection," www.asrm.org /Media/Press/genderselection.html, October 1, 2001.

9. G. Kolata, "Fertility Ethics Authority Approves Sex Selection." *New York Times*, September 28, 2001, A16.

10. M. Smith, "Gene Therapy Restores Fertility in Male Mice," *WebMD*, www.aoisvc.health.webmed.aol.com/content/article/1819.50460, January 28, 2002.

11. American Society for Reproductive Medicine, "Patient's Fact Sheet: Multiple Gestation and Multifetal Pregnancy Reduction," www.asrm .org/Patients/FactSheets/Multiple_Gestation-Fact.pdf, 1996.

12. D. Seifer, W. Dodson, R. Reindollar, and N. Santoro, "Strategies to Prevent Multiple Pregnancy During Infertility Treatment," *Contemporary OB/GYN*, 46 (February 2001): 57.

13. American Society for Reproductive Medicine, "Patient's Fact Sheet: Multiple Gestation and Multifetal Pregnancy Reduction."

14. Seifer et al., "Strategies to Prevent Multiple Pregnancies."

15. C.W. Henderson, "Research Reveals Strategies to Avoid Multiple Births," *Women's Health Weekly* (November 16, 2000): 13.

16. NewsRX.com, "Association Responds to New Report on Trends in Multiples Following Infertility Treatment," *Medical Letter on the CDC and FDA,* http://web6.infotrac.galegroup.com/itw/infomark/810/243 /20583282w6/purl=rc1_HRC_0_A63593702&dyn=9!xrn_5_0_A635937 02&bkm_9_5?sw_aep=bergen_main, July 30, 2000.

17. C. Kalb, "Should You Have Your Baby Now?" *Newsweek* 138 (August 13, 2001): 40–48.

18. National Center for Chronic Disease Prevention and Health Promotion, "1999 Assisted Reproductive Technology Success Rates," www.cdc .gov/nccdphp/drh/art.htm, 2001.

19. "Too Old to Have a Baby?" *The Lancet* 341 (February 6, 1993): 344.

20. M. Quigley, "The New Frontier of Reproductive Age," *Journal of the American Medical Association* 268 (September 9, 1992): 1320 (2).

21. J. Eisner, "Fertility and Folly," *The Gazette* (Montreal), August 20, 2001, op-ed B3.

22. J. Travis, "Dancer Gets First Ovarian-Tissue Transplant," *Science News* 156 (October 2, 1999): 212.

23. "Transplants Boost Fertility Hope," *Miami Herald Sun*, October 6, 2001, 52.

24. E. Kiely, "Ex-Wife Blocks Use of Leftover Embryos," *Pittsburgh Post-Gazette*, August 15, 2001, A1.

25. S. Schmickle, "About Stem Cells," *Minneapolis Star Tribune*, August 10, 2001, 15A.

26. T. Ackerman and B. Roth, "In Stem Cell Debate, What Comes Next?" *Houston Chronicle*, August 11, 2001, A1.

27. S. Roan, "Open Enrollment," *Los Angeles Times*, September 24, 2001, S1.

28. L. Neumeister, "Fertility Doctor Gets Seven Years in Prison," *Hackensack* (New Jersey) *Record*, October 16, 2001, A7.

29. R. Weiss, "Cloning Project Creates First Copy Cat." *Hackensack* (New Jersey) *Record*, February 15, 2002, 1.

30. J. Donn, "First Human Embryo Has Been Cloned, Scientists Say," *West Paterson* (New Jersey) *Herald News*, November 26, 2001, 1.

31. R. Weiss, "Scientist Cites Progress in Cloning of Kidneys," *Hackensack* (New Jersey) *Record*, January 30, 2002, 1.

32. Kalb, "Should You Have Your Baby Now?"

Glossary

acupuncture   A form of holistic medicine that involves piercing specific parts of the body with fine needles.

adhesion   Scar tissue occurring in the abdominal cavity, fallopian tubes, or inside the uterus. Adhesions can interfere with transport of the egg and implantation of the embryo in the uterus.

adoption   The process of legally taking a child into one's family to raise as one's own.

andrologist   A medical specialist who diagnoses and treats sperm dysfunction.

anonymous oocyte donation (AOD)   A program in which neither the egg donor nor the prospective birth parents know each other's identity.

antibody   A protective agent produced by the body's immune system in response to a foreign substance.

antigen   Any substance that induces the formation of an antibody.

antisperm antibodies   Antibodies that can attach to sperm and inhibit movement of sperm or fertilization.

artificial insemination (AI)   The process in which sperm are placed into the female reproductive tract for the purpose of producing a pregnancy.

asexual reproduction   Reproduction in which an organism produces one or more clones of itself.

assisted hatching   A procedure to facilitate hatching in which a small breach in the outer layer of the membrane surrounding the egg is made before placing the embryo in the uterus.

assisted reproductive technology (ART)   Several procedures used to bring about conception without sexual intercourse, including IUI, IVF, GIFT, and ZIFT.

asthenospermia   A condition in which there is slow-moving sperm in the seminal fluid.

azoospermia   A condition in which there are no sperm in the seminal fluid.

basal body temperature (BBT)   The temperature taken at its lowest point in the day, usually in the morning before getting out of bed.

biochemical analysis of semen   A diagnostic test that measures various chemicals in semen such as fructose.

biopsy   The removal and examination of tissue, cells, or fluids from the living body.

blastocyst   A fertilized egg that has divided into hundreds of cells over 5 days.

bromocriptine (Parlodel)   A fertility drug used to treat women whose ovulation cycles are irregular due to elevated levels of prolactin.

catheter   A tubular, flexible surgical instrument for withdrawing fluids from or introducing fluids into a body cavity.

cervical mucus   A viscous fluid plugging the opening of the cervix. Most of the time this thick mucus plug prevents sperm and bacteria from entering the womb. However, at midcycle, under the influence of estrogen, the mucus becomes thin, watery, and stringy to allow sperm to pass into the womb.

cervix   The lower section of the uterus that protrudes into the vagina and dilates during labor to allow the passage of the fetus.

chlamydia   A type of bacteria that is frequently transmitted sexually between partners or from an infected mother to her newborn child; the most common sexually transmitted bacterial disease.

chromosomes   Threads of DNA in a cell's nucleus that transmit hereditary information.

clomiphene citrate (Clomid, Serophene, Milophene)   A fertility drug that stimulates ovulation through the release of gonadotropins from the pituitary gland.

clone   A genetically identical organism.

cloning The process in which clones are established asexually, in which cells are all genetically identical to a single ancestor.

coculture A culture medium for IVF using cells taken from the woman who will receive the embryos at transfer.

conception The fertilization of a woman's egg by a man's sperm to form a zygote.

congenital Referring to conditions that are present at birth regardless of their cause.

controlled ovarian hyperstimulation (COH) *See* ovulation induction, superovulation

cryopreservation Freezing fertilized eggs or embryos after an IVF procedure for future use.

cryptorchidism An undescended testicle.

cytoplasmic transfer A procedure in which cellular material from the egg of a donor is transplanted to the egg of a woman whose embryos develop poorly. The recipient's genetic material remains.

diethylstilbestrol (DES) A synthetic estrogen (originally prescribed to prevent miscarriage) that caused malformation of the reproductive organs in some who were exposed to the drug during fetal development.

domestic adoption The adoption of an American-born child by an American couple.

donor insemination Medical substitution of the egg or sperm of the intended parents with that of a donor.

donor surrogacy A surrogate parenting arrangement in which an embryo created in vitro with the genetic material of one of the intended parents (mother or father) and donor egg or sperm is transferred to the surrogate.

ectopic pregnancy Also known as a *tubal pregnancy*, a pregnancy in which the fertilized egg implants itself outside the uterus, usually in the fallopian tubes.

electroejaculation (EEJ) A procedure in which an electric probe is placed inside the rectum against the prostate and seminal vesicles to trigger a reflex type of ejaculation.

embryo The developing baby from fertilization to the second month of pregnancy.

embryo transfer   In the IVF process, the placement of a fertilized egg back into the woman's body.

endometrial biopsy   A diagnostic procedure during which a sample of the uterine lining is collected for microscopic analysis. The biopsy results will confirm ovulation and the proper preparation of the endometrium by estrogen and progesterone stimulation.

endometriosis   A disease in which normal endometrial tissue (the lining of the uterus) grows outside of the uterus.

endometrium   The inner layer of the uterine wall that contains tubular uterine glands; the structure, thickness, and state of the endometrium undergo marked change with the menstrual cycle.

epididymis   The long, coiled tube that rests on the back side of each testicle. It transports and stores the sperm cells produced in the testes.

epididymostomy   A surgical procedure to bypass an obstruction of the epididymis.

estrogen   A female hormone produced mainly by the ovaries from puberty to menopause. It is responsible for thickening of the uterine lining during the first half of the menstrual cycle in preparation for ovulation and possible pregnancy.

fallopian tubes   A pair of ducts that pick up the egg from the ovary, where a sperm normally meets the egg to fertilize it.

falloposcopy   A diagnostic procedure that allows the visual examination of the inside of the fallopian tube.

FASIAR (follicular reduction/intraperitoneal insemination)   An insemination procedure in which a needle aspiration is used to remove some of the eggs before the sperm are flushed in.

fertility treatment   Any method or procedure used to enhance fertility or increase the likelihood of pregnancy, such as ovulation induction treatment, varicocele repair, and microsurgery to repair damaged fallopian tubes.

fertilization   The penetration of the egg by the sperm and fusion of genetic materials to result in the development of an embryo.

fetus   The developing baby from the second month of pregnancy until birth.

fimbriae   The fingerlike projections at the end of the fallopian tube nearest the ovary that capture the egg and deliver it into the tube.

follicle A fluid-filled sac in the ovary that contains an egg that is released at ovulation each month. The follicle grows to about 1 inch when it is ready to ovulate.

follicle-stimulating hormone (FSH) The pituitary hormone that stimulates follicle growth in women and sperm formation in men.

follicular phase The preovulatory phase of a woman's cycle during which the follicle grows and high estrogen levels cause the uterine lining to proliferate.

fragment removal An IVF procedure that pierces the shells of fertilized eggs to remove cellular debris.

frozen embryo transfer (FET) The replacement of cryopreserved embryo in a monitored, natural medicated hormone replacement cycle.

gamete The male and female reproductive cells—the sperm (spermatozoon) and the egg (ovum).

gamete intrafallopian transfer (GIFT) A method of assisted reproduction that involves surgically removing an egg from the ovary via laparoscopy, combining it with sperm and immediately placing the sperm/eggs into the fallopian tube, where fertilization may occur.

genetic surrogacy A surrogate parenting arrangement in which the surrogate mother is inseminated with the sperm from the male partner of the intended couple.

gestation The period of development from the time of fertilization until birth.

gestational surrogacy A surrogate parenting arrangement in which an egg is retrieved from the female of the intended couple and combined with her male partner's sperm, and the resulting embryo is implanted in the surrogate.

GnRH analogs (Lupron, Synarel, Zoladex) A fertility drug used to treat women who ovulate prematurely during hMG treatment.

gonadotropin-releasing hormone (**GnRH**) (Factrel, Lutrepulse) The hormone produced and released by the hypothalamus that controls the pituitary gland's production and release of gonadotropins.

gonadotropins The hormones produced by the pituitary gland that control reproductive function, such as follicle-stimulating hormone (FSH) and luteinizing hormone (LH).

gonorrhea   A sexually transmitted infection that causes inflammation of the mucous membrane and can also lead to infertility. It is caused by *Neisseria gonococcus*, a bacteria.

gynecologist   A doctor who specializes in the diseases and routine physical care of the reproductive system of women.

hamster test   A test of sperm's ability to penetrate a hamster egg that has been stripped of the zona pellucida (outer membrane). Also called *sperm penetration assay* (SPA).

hemizona assay   A laboratory test of sperm's ability to penetrate into a human egg; first the egg is split in half, and then one-half is tested against the male's sperm and the other half against sperm from a fertile man.

higher-order multiples   Three or more fetuses in one pregnancy.

homeopathy   A system of medical treatment based on the use of small quantities of a substance that in larger doses produces symptoms similar to the disease being treated.

hormone   A substance, produced by an endocrine gland, that travels through the bloodstream to a specific organ, where it exerts its effect.

hostile mucus   Cervical mucus that impedes the natural progress of sperm through the cervical canal.

human chorionic gonadotropin (hCG) (Perganyl)   A fertility drug used to stimulate the follicle to release the egg.

human menopausal gonadotropin (hMG) (Pergonal, Humegon, Repronex)   A fertility drug that stimulates the ovaries to induce ovulation.

human zona pellucida binding test   A test that measures the ability of sperm to bind to the zona pellucida (outer covering) of the egg.

hypo-osmotic swelling test   A test that assesses the sperm membrane for structural integrity.

hysterosalpingogram (HSG)   A radiographic procedure in which a special dye is injected into the uterus to illustrate the inner contour of the uterus and degree of openness (patency) of the fallopian tubes.

hysteroscopy   Examination of the inner cavity of the uterus through a fiberoptic telescope inserted through the vagina and cervical canal.

ICSI   *See* intracytoplasmic sperm injection

idiopathic infertility A diagnosis indicating no cause of infertility can be identified in either partner, yet pregnancy does not ensue.

implantation Attachment of the fertilized egg to the uterine lining, usually occurring 5 to 7 days after ovulation.

impotence Complete or partial inability of a man to achieve an erection or ejaculation.

in utero While in the uterus during early development.

in vitro Outside the human body.

in vitro fertilization (IVF) A method of assisted reproduction that involves surgically removing eggs from the ovary with a long needle (by ultrasound-guided retrieval) after ovulation induction, combining it with sperm in a petri dish, and, after fertilization, replacing the resulting embryo(s) in the woman's uterus. Also called *test tube baby* and *test tube fertilization*.

in vitro maturation A technique of assisted reproduction technology that involves the intentional retrieval of oocytes before they are fully mature with subsequent growth in the laboratory.

in vivo Within the body.

incompetent cervix A cervix with the inability to remain closed throughout an entire pregnancy; a frequent cause of premature birth.

infertility The inability of a couple to achieve a pregnancy or to carry a pregnancy to term after 1 year of unprotected intercourse or the inability of the woman to carry a pregnancy to live birth. *Primary infertility* indicates that the patient has never achieved a pregnancy, whereas *secondary infertility* denotes that a previous pregnancy was achieved, regardless of outcome.

international adoption The adoption by an American couple of a child who was born in a country other than the United States.

intracervical insemination (ICI) Artificial insemination of sperm into the cervical canal.

intracytoplasmic sperm injection (ICSI) A micromanipulation technique requiring the penetration of the zona pellucida and oolemma (outer coatings) of the egg with a sharp glass needle through which a single, selected sperm is introduced directly into the cytoplasm (outside of the egg).

intratubal insemination (ITI) Artificial insemination of sperm, which have been washed free of seminal fluid, into the fallopian tubes.

intrauterine insemination (IUI)   Artificial insemination of sperm, which have been washed free of seminal fluid, into the uterine cavity.

Kallmann's syndrome   A condition characterized by infantile sexual development and an inability to smell. Since the pituitary cannot produce LH and FSH, the woman must take hormone supplements to achieve puberty, to maintain secondary sex characteristics, and to achieve fertility.

Klinefelter's syndrome   A chromosome abnormality with a 47 XXY pattern, which prevents normal male sexual development and causes reversible infertility due to the presence of an extra female (X) chromosome. These men present with azoospermia.

laparoscopy   A minor surgical procedure that allows visualization of the inside of the abdomen or pelvis using a special thin telescope called a *laparoscope*.

Leydig cells   The cells in the testicles that make testosterone.

LH surge   The sudden release of luteinizing hormone (LH) that causes the follicle to release a mature egg.

local anesthesia   Anesthetic medication usually injected into the tissue to cause a small region of numbness.

luteal phase   Postovulatory phase of a woman's cycle; the corpus luteum produces progesterone, which in turn causes the uterine lining to secrete substances to support the implantation and growth of the early embryo.

luteal phase defect (LPD)   Inadequate function of the corpus luteum that may prevent a fertilized egg from implanting in the uterus or may lead to early pregnancy loss.

luteinizing hormone (LH)   The hormone that normally triggers ovulation and stimulates the corpus luteum to secrete progesterone; produced and released by the pituitary gland. In the male, it stimulates testosterone production.

luteinizing hormone surge   The sharp rise in the blood level of LH that triggers ovulation.

male factor infertility or **male infertility**   Infertility caused by a problem in the male partner.

microinjection fallopian transfer (MIFT)   A technique similar to GIFT and ZIFT that may be used in lieu of in vitro fertilization for women with patent (clear and open) tubes. After egg retrieval, the eggs are mixed with sperm and then immediately injected through into the woman's fallopian tubes for in vivo fertilization.

microsurgical epididymal sperm aspiration (MESA) A technique using microsurgery to remove sperm from the epididymis for use in in vitro fertilization, often with ICSI.

miscarriage The spontaneous loss of an embryo or fetus from the womb. Also called *spontaneous abortion*.

mitochondria A component of egg cytoplasm that fuels many of its functions.

morphology The shape of sperm as studied in a semen analysis.

motility The measurement of motion and forward progression of sperm in a semen analysis.

mucus A viscid slippery secretion that is produced by mucous membranes that it moistens and protects.

natural hormones Compounded hormones made in a lab that are bio-identical to the body's natural hormones.

oligospermia An abnormally low number of sperm in the ejaculate of the male.

oocyte The immature ovum, the unfertilized female gamete or sex cell (egg) produced in the ovaries each month, that contains the genetic information to be transmitted by the female.

oocyte retrieval A surgical procedure to collect the eggs contained within the ovarian follicles, either via laparoscopic or ultrasound-guided follicular aspiration through which a needle is inserted into the follicle and the fluid and egg are aspirated into the needle and then placed into a culture medium–filled dish.

ovarian hyperstimulation syndrome A condition that can occur when women use ovarian stimulation medications.

ovaries The sexual glands of the female that produce the hormones estrogen and progesterone and in which the ova are developed.

ovulation The release of a mature egg from the ovarian follicle; usually occurs on approximately day 14 of a normal 28-day menstrual cycle.

ovulation induction (OI) Pharmacological stimulation of the ovaries, generally with gonadotropins and/or clomiphene citrate, with the objective of stimulating the development of multiple follicles and hence multiple eggs. Also called *controlled ovarian hyperstimulation*.

pathology   The structural and functional effects of disease on the body (or the study of such).

pelvic inflammatory disease (PID)   An infection of the pelvic organs that causes severe illness, high fever, and extreme pain. PID may lead to tubal blockage and pelvic adhesions.

penis   The male organ of sexual intercourse.

percutaneous epididymal sperm aspiration (PESA)   A procedure in which a small needle is passed directly into the head of the epididymis and fluid is aspirated. Any sperm found are used in conjunction with in vitro fertilization with ICSI.

Pergonal (hMG)   A substance made from the luteinizing and follicle-stimulating hormones recovered from postmenopausal women's urine that is used to induce multiple ovulation in various fertility treatments.

perinatologist   A doctor specializing in treating the fetus/baby and mother during pregnancy, labor, and delivery, particularly when the mother and/or baby are at a high risk for complications.

peroxidase staining   A diagnostic technique that differentiates white blood cells from immature sperm to assess for possible infection.

polycystic ovarian syndrome (PCOS)   A condition found among women who do not ovulate, characterized by multiple ovarian cysts and increased androgen production.

postcoital test (PCT)   A microscopic examination of the cervical mucus performed several hours after intercourse to detect sperm-mucus interaction problems, the presence of sperm antibodies, and the quality of the cervical mucus.

pregnancy reduction   *See* selective reduction

preimplantation diagnosis (PGD)   A technique using biopsy in which a single cell is removed from an embryo and assessed for chromosomal abnormality.

primary infertility (PI)   Refers to those struggling with infertility without ever having conceived. Popular usage has been extended to include those who have conceived but have not had a live birth.

progesterone   An ovarian hormone secreted by the corpus luteum during the second half of the menstrual cycle after ovulation has occurred; also produced by the placenta during pregnancy.

regional anesthetic   *See* local anesthesia

reproductive endocrinologist (RE)   A medical specialist combining obstetrics and gynecology with endocrinology to treat reproductive disorders.

retrograde ejaculation   Ejaculation backward into the bladder instead of forward through the urethra.

scrotum   The sac containing the testicles, epididymis, and vas deferens.

secondary infertility (SI)   The inability of a couple to achieve a second pregnancy. This strict medical definition includes couples for whom the pregnancy did not go to term. The common vernacular, however, refers to a couple who has one biological child (or more) but is unable to conceive another.

selective reduction   An intentional reduction in the number of fetuses in women with multifetal gestation; also called *pregnancy reduction*.

semen   The fluid containing sperm and secretions from the testicles, prostate, and seminal vesicles that is expelled during ejaculation.

semen analysis (SA)   A laboratory test used to assess semen quality: sperm quantity, concentration, morphology (form), and motility. In addition, it measures semen volume and whether white blood cells are present, indicating an infection.

semen culture   A laboratory test that checks for bacteria that may cause genital infection.

sexually transmitted disease (STD)   A disease caused by an infectious agent transmitted during sex.

sonogram   A technique that uses high-frequency sound waves for creating an image of internal body parts.

sonohysterography (SHG)   An ultrasound-monitored procedure used to detect abnormalities of the uterus and fallopian tubes or tubal blockage.

sperm   The male gamete or sex cell that contains the genetic information to be transmitted by the male; also known as *spermatozoon* (plural: *spermatozoa*).

sperm bank   A place where sperm are kept frozen in liquid nitrogen for later use in artificial insemination or IVF.

sperm chromatin structure assay (SCSA)   A test that can detect the percentage of sperm with DNA damage.

sperm count (density) The number of sperm in ejaculate. Also called *sperm concentration* or *sperm density* and given as the number of sperm per milliliter.

sperm morphology The shape or form of the sperm cells.

sperm motility The quality of sperm cells demonstrating any type of movement.

sperm penetration assay (SPA) *See* hamster test

sperm viability Whether or not the sperm are alive.

sperm washing A laboratory technique for separating sperm from semen, and separating motile sperm from nonmotile sperm, for use in assisted reproduction.

spermicide An agent that kills sperm.

spinnbarkeit The cervical mucus that becomes more profuse, thinner, wetter, stretchier, and clearer just before ovulation; also called *spinn*.

spontaneous miscarriage A pregnancy ending in miscarriage with or without an operative procedure.

stem cells The master cells of the body that give rise to other cells needed for growth and maintenance.

sterility An irreversible condition that prevents conception.

strict morphology determination A laboratory test that gives detailed examination of sperm shapes.

superovulation Stimulation of multiple ovulation with fertility drugs; also known as *controlled ovarian hyperstimulation* (COH).

surrogate A woman who is employed, for a fee or not, by the intended parents to carry a child through pregnancy and delivery.

teratospermia A condition in which there is abnormally shaped sperm in the seminal fluid.

testes or **testicles** The two male sexual glands contained in the scrotum. They produce the male hormone testosterone and the male reproductive cells (sperm).

testicular biopsy A minor surgical procedure used to take a small sample of testicular tissue for microscopic examination; a test used to diagnose male fertility problems when no other means is available (because the biopsy procedure itself may cause testicular damage).

testicular enzyme defect   A congenital enzyme defect that prevents the testes from responding to hormonal stimulation; will result in oligospermia or azoospermia.

testicular sperm aspiration (TESA)   A needle biopsy of the testicle used to obtain small amounts of sperm. A small incision is made in the scrotal skin and a spring-loaded needle is inserted through the testicle.

testicular sperm extraction (TESE)   An open biopsy in which a small piece of testicular tissue is removed through a skin incision. The tissue is placed in culture media and separated into tiny pieces. Sperm are released from within the seminiferous tubules where they are produced and are then extracted from the surrounding testicular tissue.

testicular stress pattern   A semen analysis result showing depressed sperm production, poor sperm motility, and poor sperm morphology. The pattern is consistent with secondary testicular failure or illness.

transuterine fallopian transfer (TUFT)   The placement of an embryo inside the fallopian tube after in vitro fertilization.

tubal embryo transfer (TET)   The placement of an embryo inside the fallopian tube after in vitro fertilization.

tubal ligation reversal   A surgical procedure to reverse female sterilization due to surgically cut fallopian tubes.

tubal pregnancy   *See* ectoptic pregnancy

Turner's syndrome   A genetic defect contributing to female fertility problems.

ultrasound   *See* sonogram

undescended testicles   The failure of the testicles to descend from the abdominal cavity into the scrotum by 1 year of age; also called *cryptorchidism*. If not repaired by age 6, it may result in permanent fertility loss.

unexplained infertility   A diagnosis of exclusion, once both partners have been evaluated, that indicates that the reasons for infertility cannot be determined.

urethra   The tube through which urine from the bladder is expelled.

urologist   A surgeon who specializes in the treatment of disorders of the urinary tract in men and women and the reproductive tract in men.

uterus   The reproductive organ that houses, protects, and nourishes the developing embryo/fetus. It is a hollow, muscular structure that is part of the female reproductive tract and is the source of a woman's menses.

vagina   The female organ of sexual intercourse; the birth canal.

varicocele   Varicose veins in the scrotum. The resulting swollen vessels surrounding the testicles create a pool of stagnant blood, which elevates the scrotal temperature. A major cause of male infertility.

varicocelectomy   A surgical repair of a varicocele.

vas deferens   The pair of thick-walled tubes through which the sperm move from the epididymis to the ejaculatory duct in the prostate. These tubes are severed during a vasectomy performed for birth control.

vasectomy   The surgical separation of both vas deferens, used for birth control/sterilization.

vasogram   An x ray of the vas deferens to see whether it is blocked.

vital staining   A laboratory test that determines numbers of living and dead sperm.

waiting-child adoption   Adoption of an older and often hard-to-place child from the social services system.

zygote   An egg that has been fertilized but not yet divided.

zygote intrafallopian transfer (ZIFT)   In vitro fertilization with a transfer of the zygote into the fallopian tube.

Index

A

Acupuncture, 102–109

Adalat (nifedipine), 91

Adaptogens, defined, 114

Adoption

  cautionary advice on, 203–207

  domestic, 191

  empowered couples and,
    195–198, 200

  as happy ending, 200–203

  international, 191–192

  questions to ask about, 199

  resource referrals, 194

  statistics on, 190

  waiting-child, 192–193, 195

Age

  controversy over, 264–266

  ethical debates over, 267–268

  female fertility and, 10–12

  female infertility testing and, 56–59

  male fertility and, 30–31

  medical issues with, 267

  practical concerns over, 267

Aiman, James, 15

Alcohol, 84, 90

American Association of Clinical
    Endocrinologists, 39

American Board of Medical
    Specialties, 39

American Society for Reproductive
    Medicine (ASRM), 12, 37, 40, 47,
    52, 59, 91, 92, 131, 132, 151,
    251–252, 257, 258, 261, 266

Americans with Disabilities Act
    (ADA), 280

Ampulla, defined, 5

Anatomy

  female, 3–5

  male, 6–7

Andrologists, 38–39

Antisperm antibodies, 31–32, 141

Applebaum, Dr. Michael, 62

Aristotle, 17

Aromatherapy, 231–232

Artificial insemination

  Angela's story, 148–150

  description of, 145–150

  parentage options with, 152

Asch, Ricardo, 19

Assisted reproductive technology (ART)

  artificial insemination, 145–150

  in vitro fertilization, 144, 150–167,
    168–169

  recent advances in, 246–255

  traditional Chinese medicine and,
    104–107

Asthenospermia, 27

Azoospermia, 27, 32

B

Baby showers, 218–219

Basal body temperature (BBT) reading, 75–77

Belgrade, Dr. Miles, 103

Benoff, Dr. Susan, 91

Benson, Dr. Herbert, 240

Berger, Dr. Gary, 86, 138–39

Berry, Martin, 18

Biochemical pregnancy, 9

Biofeedback, 230–231

Blackwell, Dr. Keith, 281

Blastocyst, defined, 145

Blum, Melanie, 274–276

Boldt, Dr. Jeffrey, 269

Boxer shorts versus briefs, 30, 93

Brackett, Dr. Nancy, 157

Bradford, Hannah, 102–104, 108

Breathing, deep, 228–229

Bromocriptine (Parlodel), 135

Brown, Louise, 151, 283

Bush, President George W., 274

C

Caffeine, 84, 89–90

Cameron, Myra, 232

Cancer
    fertility drugs and, 137
    male infertility and, 29, 55
    women with, 269–270, 271

Caplan, Arthur, 151

Carr, Elizabeth Jordan, 151

Causes of female infertility
    age, 10–12, 21
    endometriosis, 21, 22, 139–140
    ovulatory disorders, 21, 22–23
    repeat miscarriages, 23–25, 140
    tubal factors, 21–22, 138

unexplained, 21
    uterine problems, 137–138

Causes of male infertility
    age, 30–31
    anatomical defects, 26, 28–29
    blocked tube, 26, 28–29
    hormonal factors, 26, 29
    infections, 26, 27
    sperm problems, 25
    varicoceles, 26–27

Cervical mucus monitoring, 77–78

Cervix
    defined, 3
    illustrations of, 4, 5
    incompetent, 140

Childless by Choice, 210

Childless lifestyle
    as option, 207
    social reengineering and, 209–212
    stages of grief and, 208–209

Cigarette smoking, 45, 87, 88–89

Clement, Brian, 84

Clomid, 10, 11, 68, 69, 98, 134, 148, 149, 150, 168

Clomiphene citrate (Clomid, Serophene, Milophene), 29, 41, 105, 134, 136, 257

Clomiphene citrate challenge test, 60

Cloning debate, 281–283

Coculturing, 265

Cognitive restructuring, 233–235

Cohen, Dr. Jacques, 247, 253

Cold medicine, 80

Combined infertility, 31–32

Commutes, long, 93

Complementary and alternative medicine (CAM)
    acupuncture, 102–109
    herbal remedies, 113–120

holistic medicine, 96–97
homeopathy, 109–112
natural hormone balancing, 97–102
naturopathic physicians, 124–126
physical therapy, 120–121
total body health, 126–129
Wurn technique, 122–124
Computer monitors, 87
Conception
    brief biology lesson on, 2
    female's role, 3–5
    male's role, 5–7
Conkling, Winifred, 90
Corsello, Dr. Serafina, 207–208, 209, 210
Corson, Dr. Stephen, 64–65
Cough medicine, 80
Counseling, 242–244
Cowper's glands, defined, 7
Crinone, 135

D

Daniluk, Dr. Judith, 221
Degnan, Dr. Peter, 82–84, 94
Delury, Anna, 236
Depression, 208, 240–242
Diagnosis
    as difficult process, 35–36
    emotional aspect of, 40–41
    female workup, 56–66
    finding a doctor, 36–40
    male workup, 42–55
    marital and sexual history, 41–42
    Melinda's story, 67–71
    of repeat miscarriages, 8, 66–67
Diagnostic tests for female. *See also*
    Medical treatment of females
    age and, 56–59
    falloposcopy, 65–66
    hormone testing, 59–60

hysterosalpingogram (HSG), 17, 57,
    58, 61–62, 67
hysteroscopy, 62–63, 69
laparoscopy, 63–65, 69
postcoital test, 56, 58, 65
sonohysterography (SHG), 57, 62
ultrasound exams, 60–61
Diagnostic tests for male. *See also*
    Medical treatment of males
    importance of, 42–44
    medical history and, 44–45
    physical exam and, 45–46
    sperm analysis, 46–54
    testes biopsy, 54, 156–157
    ultrasound exam, 54
    vasography, 54
Diaphragm breathing, 228–229
Diet, 81–85
Diethylstilbestrol (DES), 29, 44, 56
Digby, Sir Kenelm, 18
Dion, Celine, 279
Dipasquale, Dr. Robin, 113–116
Directory of Medical Specialists, 39
Doctors
    infertility specialists, 36–40
    naturopathic physicians, 124–126
Domar, Dr. Alice, 233–234, 240
Donor insemination
    anonymous donors, 175–177
    cost of, 176–177
    description of, 173–175
    ethical issues, 177–178
    nonanonymous donors, 178–180
Donor surrogacy, 182
Douching, 81
Doyle, Kate, 276
Driving, 93
Drugs
    illicit, 45, 90–91
    medical history and, 44, 45

Drugs, fertility
    commonly used, 134–135
    ovulatory disorders and, 132–134
    risks of, 135–137
Dumesic, Dr. Daniel A., 158

E

Echinacea, 119
Ectopic pregnancy, 137
Edwards, Dr. Robert, 150, 151
Eisner, Jane, 267
Ejaculation, retrograde
    artificial insemination and,
        145–150
    defined, 28
    treatment for, 141–142
Electroejaculation (EEJ), 156–157
Embryo, defined, 145
Embryo coculture, 265
Embryo transfer, 161–163
Embryos, leftover
    court battles over, 272–273
    cryopreservation of, 166–167
    protecting, 274–276
    for research, 273–274
Endometrial biopsy, 67
Endometriosis
    as cause of infertility, 21, 22
    laparoscopy and, 65
    medical treatment for, 139–140, 153
Environmental toxins, 85–88
Epididymostomy, 143
Eustachio, Bartolomeo, 18
Exercise, 94–95

F

Fallopian tube disorders
    as cause of infertility, 21–22
    medical treatment for, 138, 153

Fallopian tubes
    damaged, 14, 21–22
    defined, 4
    illustration of, 5
Falloposcopy, 65–66
False unicorn root, 115
FASIAR procedure, 147
Fecundity, 30
Female infertility. *See also* Miscarriages,
        repeat
    causes of, 21–23
    defined, 2
    repeat miscarriages, 8, 23–25
    smoking and, 88
Female infertility treatments. *See*
        Complementary and alternative
        medicine; Medical treatment of
        females
Female reproductive system, 3–5
Female workup
    diagnostic tests, 56–66
    physical exam, 56
    for repeat miscarriages, 66–67
    story about, 67–71
Fertile Garden herbal formula, 116–117
Fertility drugs
    commonly used, 134–135
    ovulatory disorders and, 132–134
    risks of, 135–137
Fertility preservation
    cautious optimism for, 271–272
    freezing egg-containing ovarian
        tissue, 269, 270
    freezing eggs, 269–270
    ovarian implant, 269, 270–271
Fertility specialists
    finding, 36–39
    questions to ask, 39–40
Fertility studies, history of, 15–20
Fimbriae, defined, 4
Folic acid, 84

Follicle-stimulating hormone (FSH)
    defined, 3, 92, 99, 133
    as fertility drug treatment, 133, 134
    hormone testing and, 45, 57, 59–60
    intrauterine insemination (IUI)
        and, 146
    Kallmann's syndrome and, 32
    in the male, 29
    polycystic ovary syndrome and, 23
Follistim, 60, 98, 134, 148, 152, 168
Food and fertility, 81–85, 86
Food Guide Pyramid, 85, 86
Ford, Dr. Chris, 30
Fourcroy, Dr. Jean, 38, 42, 43, 44, 45,
    46, 47, 49, 54, 142, 160
Freezing eggs, 269–270
FSH. *See* Follicle-stimulating hormone

G

Gamete, defined, 145
Gamete intrafallopian transfer (GIFT),
    19–20, 162, 163, 165, 172
Genetic conditions, 32
Genetic diagnosis
    preimplantation, 250–252
    scanning IVF embryos for, 255
Gestational surrogacy, 181
Gibbs, Peter, 195–196, 198, 199, 200
Gindoff, Dr. Paul R., 40, 41, 56–59,
    247, 249, 260, 265, 271
Ginkgo, 119
Glucose intolerance, 133
GnRH. *See* Gonadotropin-releasing
    hormone
GnRH analogs, 135, 271
Goldstein, Dr. Marc, 43, 44, 93,
    142, 157
Gonadotropin-releasing hormone
    (GnRH), 29, 92, 134–135
Gonadotropins, 60, 257

Goodman, Dr. Neil F., 264, 268
Grant, Theresa Venet, 13, 36, 37, 42
Grifo, Dr. James, 252
Guaifenesin, 80
Guzick, Dr. David S., 32, 146

H

Habana, Antonia, 166
Hahnemann, Dr. Samuel, 109, 110
Harris , Ron, 177
Harvey, William, 18
Health insurance
    controversy over, 276–277
    facts about, 277–280
    infertility as disability, 280–281
    multiple births and, 261–263, 277
Herbal remedies
    for anxiety, 113–114
    Fertile Garden formula, 116–117
    for liver function, 116
    for men, 117–118
    for menstrual dysfunction, 115–116
    for ovarian dysfunction, 115
    for stress, 114
    unregulated, 120
    warnings regarding, 118–119
Hertwig, Oscar, 18
Higher-order multiples
    clinic success rates and, 261
    defined, 257
    fertility drugs and, 136, 257
    insurance reform and, 261–263, 277
    medical complications of, 257–258
    patient education and, 263–264
    reduction strategies, 258–260
    statistics on, 258
Hippocrates, 15–17
History of fertility studies, 15–20
Holistic medicine, 96–97
Hollister, Margaret, 262

Homeopathy, 109–112

Hormone balancing, natural, 97–102

Hormone testing, 45, 59–60

Horstman, Judith, 108

Huhner, Max, 19

Human chorionic gonadotropin (hCG), 134, 136, 153

Human cloning, 281–283

Human zona pellucida binding tests, 53

Hunter, John, 18

Hypoglycemics, 133

Hysterosalpingogram, 17, 57, 58, 61–62, 67

Hysteroscopy, 62–63, 69

I

Idiopathic infertility, 32–33

Imagery, mental, 229

Impotence
  infertility versus, 43
  smoking and, 89

In vitro, defined, 145

In vitro fertilization (IVF)
  best method of, 165–166
  blastocyst culture and transfer, 161–162, 248–249
  defined, 19, 150
  extra embryos and, 166–167, 272–276
  female diagnostic testing and, 57–58
  first "test tube" baby, 19, 150–151, 283
  history of, 150–152
  ovary-stimulating drugs and, 154
  preimplantation genetic diagnosis (PGD) and, 250–252
  six steps of, 152–163
  success rates, 164
  Traci's story, 168–169
  traditional Chinese medicine (TCM) and, 104–107
  twenty-four ways to make a baby and, 171–172

In vivo, defined, 145

Infertility
  age and, 10–12, 30–31, 264–268
  causes of, 20–32
  combined, 31–32
  defined, 2
  facts about, 8–9
  female, 21–25
  idiopathic, 32–33
  insurance and, 261–263, 276–281
  male, 6, 25–31
  population affected by, 13–15
  possibility of, 33–34
  sterility versus, 1

Infertility options
  adoption, 190–207
  donor eggs/sperm, 173–180
  nonparenting, 207–212
  surrogate parenting, 181–190

Infertility treatments. *See* Complementary and alternative medicine; Medical treatment of females; Medical treatment of males

Insensitive questions, 218

Insurance
  controversy over, 276–277
  facts about, 277–280
  infertility as disability, 280–281
  multiple births and, 261–263, 277

Intercourse, timed
  Clara and José's story, 82–83
  guidelines for, 79–80

International adoptions, 191–192

Intracytoplasmic sperm injection (ICSI), 53, 158–160, 171

Intrauterine insemination (IUI), defined, 145–147

Irvine, Steward, 15
Iyengar, B.K.S., 236, 239

J

Jacobsen, Rune, 55

K

Kallmann's syndrome, 32
Kanatsu-Shinohara, Mito, 256
Kearns, Dr. Clifford, 110–112
Klinefelter's syndrome, 32
Koop, C. Everett, 223
Kramer, Erin, 217, 219
Kübler-Ross, Elisabeth, 208

L

Landesman, Peter, 50, 220
Laparoscopy, 63–65, 69
Lasater, Judith Hanson, 239
Lauersen, Dr. Niels, 279
Leeuwenhoek, Antonie van, 18
Leydig cells, 27
Licorice, 114
Lifestyle habits
    alcohol, 84, 90
    caffeine, 84, 89–90
    drugs, 45, 90–91
    environmental toxins, 85–88
    exercise, 94–95
    nutrition, 81–85
    rising body heat, 93
    smoking, 45, 87, 88–89
    weight loss or gain, 91–92
Lobo, Dr. Rogerio A., 233
Luteinizing hormone (LH)
    defined, 4, 92, 99
    female hormone testing and, 59, 60

Kallmann's syndrome and, 32
in males, 29

M

MacNab, Dr. Tracy, 220
Madara, Edward, 224, 225
Madden, Dr. James, 259–260, 261,
    262, 263
Madonna, 264
Male infertility. *See also* Male
    workup
    acupuncture for, 104
    age and, 30–31
    causes of, 25–31, 86
    chromosome linked to, 32, 160
    defined, 6
    herbal remedy for, 117–118
    medical treatment for, 141–144
    smoking and, 88–89
    sperm analysis and, 46–54
Male role in conception, 6–7
Male workup. *See also* Medical treat-
    ment of males
    importance of, 43–44
    medical history, 44–45
    physical exam, 45–46
    sperm analysis, 46–54
    sperm deficiency testing, 42
    sperm quality and cancer, 29, 55
    ultrasound for, 54
Marital and sexual history, 41–42
Marital problems, 220–223
McClamrock, Dr. Howard D., 88
McNamee, Dr. Philip, 80
Medical history
    in female workup, 56
    in male workup, 44–45
Medical terms/vocabulary, 2–7,
    27, 145

Medical treatment of females. *See also*
    Assisted reproductive technology;
    Female workup
  for endometriosis, 139–140
  fertility drug treatment, 133–137
  for ovulatory disorders, 132–133
  for recurrent miscarriage, 140
  for tubal disorders, 137
  tubal ligation reversals, 138–139
  for uterine problems, 137–138
Medical treatment of males. *See also*
    Assisted reproductive technology;
    Male workup
  advances in, 255–257
  medication, 141
  for obstruction, 143
  for retrograde ejaculation, 141–142
  sperm abnormalities and, 141
  for varicoceles, 142–143
  vasectomy reversal, 143–144
Menstrual cycle
  importance of, 3
  in medical history, 56, 58
  uterus and, 5
Menstrual dysfunction
  endometriosis and, 22, 139–140
  herbs for, 115–116
  ovulatory disorders and, 22–23, 132
  traditional Chinese medicine (TCM)
    for, 105
Menstrual period tracking
  basal body temperature (BBT) read-
    ing, 75–77
  cervical mucus monitoring, 77–78
  defined, 73–75
Metformin, 133
Mikesell, Dr. Susan G., 30
Mind-body connection
  Ann's story, 214–216
  communication with spouse, 220–223
  counseling, 242–244

depression, 208, 240–242
family and friends, 217–219
infertility and, 213–214
men's self-esteem, 216
relaxation techniques, 227–240
stress, 225–227
support groups, 223–225
Miscarriages, repeat
  diagnosis of, 66–67
  environmental toxins and, 86–87
  folic acid and, 84
  as infertility, 8
  Penny's story, 24–25
  reasons for, 23–25
  treatment for, 140
Mittleschmerz, 42
Molnar, Dr. Bela, 47
Multiple births
  clinic success rates and, 261
  fertility drugs and, 136, 257
  insurance reform and, 261–263, 277
  medical complications of, 257–258
  patient education and, 263–264
  reduction strategies, 258–260
  statistics on, 258
Murphy, Eileen, 192–193, 195

N

Nasseri, Dr. Ali, 161
National Mental Health
    Association, 211
Natural hormone balancing, 97–102
Ni, Dr. Daoshing, 104, 113
Nifedipine, 91
No Kidding! website, 210
Nonparenting
  as option, 207
  social reengineering and, 209–212
  stages of grief and, 208–209
Nutrition, 81–85

O

Oktay, Dr. Kutluk, 270, 271

Older-age pregnancies
    controversy over, 264–266
    ethical debates over, 267–268
    female fertility and age, 10–12
    infertility testing and age, 56–59
    male fertility and age, 30–31
    medical issues with, 267
    practical concerns over, 267

Oligospermia, defined, 27

Oocyte, defined, 145

Ovarian hyperstimulation syndrome,
    135–136

Ovarian implant, 269, 270–271

Ovaries
    defined, 3
    illustrations of, 4, 5

Ovulation, defined, 3, 74

Ovulation kits, 78–79

Ovulatory disorders
    description of, 21, 22–23
    herbs for, 115
    medical treatment for, 132–137

P

Page, Dr. David, 160

Palermo, Dr. Gianpiero, 159

Palter, Dr. Steven, 165

Pan, Dr. John, 96–97

Parlodel (bromocriptine), 135

Pelvic inflammatory disease (PID), 22, 138

Peony (bai shao), 115

Pergonal, 98, 134, 152

Period tracking
    basal body temperature (BBT)
        reading, 75–77
    cervical mucus monitoring, 77–78
    defined, 73–75

Perloe, Dr. Mark, 37, 38, 248, 249,
    255, 256, 265, 271

Petak, Dr. Steven, 1

Peterson, Lisa Rivo, 223

Physical exam
    for females, 56
    for males, 45–46

Physical therapy
    myofascial release, 120–121
    Wurn Technique, 122–124

Pluta, Nataly, 120–121

Polycystic ovary syndrome (PCOS)
    Angela's story, 148–150
    description of, 10, 23
    treatment for, 132–133

Postcoital test, 56, 58, 65

Prayer, 232–233

Preimplantation genetic diagnosis
    (PGD), 250–252

Primary infertility, 8

Procardia (nifedipine), 91

Progesterone
    role of, 5, 99, 133–134
    as treatment, 101, 135

Prostate exam, 46

Prostate gland, defined, 7

Pycnogenol herbal supplement, 117–118

R

Ravnikar, Dr. Veronica, 23, 35, 36

Relaxation techniques
    aromatherapy, 231–232
    biofeedback, 230–231
    cognitive restructuring, 233–235
    deep breathing, 228–229
    mental imagery, 229
    prayer, 232–233
    progressive muscle relaxation, 230
    yoga, 235–239

Reproductive system
    female, 3–5
    male, 6–7

Research on assisted reproductive technology (ART)
  advances in ART, 246–247
  assisted hatching, 247
  blastocyst culture and transfer, 161–162, 248–249
  cytoplasmic transfer, 252–255
  fragment removal, 247–248
  preimplantation diagnosis (PGD), 250–252
  statistics on fertility procedures, 245–246
RESOLVE
  executive director of, 262
  Physician Referral List, 39
  support groups, 223, 224
  Web site, 243
Retrograde ejaculation
  artificial insemination and, 145–150
  defined, 28
  treatment for, 141–142
Roseff, Dr. Scott, 117, 118
Rosenthal, Dr. Jane, 242, 243
Rosenwaks, Dr. Zev, 264

S

Sable, Dr. David, 253, 254, 255
Sachdev, Dr. Rahul, 227
St. John's wort, 119
Sarandon, Susan, 264
Schlank, Christina, 278, 280
Schlegel, Dr. Peter, 43, 44, 142, 157
Scrotal temperatures, 93
Scrotum, defined, 7
Seaman, Dr. Eric, 141–142, 157
Secondary infertility, 8, 9
Semen, defined, 3. *See also* Sperm analysis
Seminal vesicles, defined, 7

Septuplets, 257. *See also* Multiple births
Sexual history, 41–42
Sexually transmitted diseases, 14, 22, 27, 44, 56, 138
Seymour, Jane, 264
Shrybman, Jimmy, 182–184, 185
Shu, Dr. Mengda, 104, 105, 107
Sigmund, Karl, 19
Silber, Dr. Sherman, 9, 11, 160
Sills, Dr. Eric Scott, 147, 155, 164, 170, 171, 174
Sims, J. Marion, 18
Skakkebaek, Niels, 15
Smoak, Dr. Randolph, 89
Smoking, 45, 87, 88–89
Social reengineering, 209–212
Somers, Wendy, 176
Sonohysterography (SHG), 57, 62
Soules, Dr. Michael, 12
Spallanzani, Lazzarro, 18
Sperm
  abnormally shaped, 17, 25, 48
  artificial insemination and, 145–150
  in vitro fertilization procedures and, 155–160
  male anatomy and, 5–7
  male infertility and, 6
  teamwork, 8
Sperm analysis
  advances in, 255–256
  description of, 46–48
  further testing after, 54
  giving sperm, 50
  Jake's story, 52–53
  Karen and Rick's story, 51
  as numbers game, 49–50
  optional sperm tests, 51–53
  testicular cancer and, 55
Sperm counts, global fall in, 15

Spinnbarkeit mucus, 77, 79

Spontaneous abortions, 8

Stem cell research, 273–274

Steptoe, Dr. Patrick, 150, 151

Steroids, 95

Stress and infertility, 225–227

Stress management
    aromatherapy, 231–232
    biofeedback, 230–231
    cognitive restructuring, 233–235
    deep breathing, 228–229
    mental imagery, 229
    prayer, 232–233
    progressive muscle relaxation, 230
    yoga, 235–239

Sullivan, Mary, 204–207

Support groups, 223–225

Surrogacy
    basic types of, 181–182
    benefits of, 182–183
    as controversial issue, 184
    cost of, 185–186
    finding a surrogate, 184–185
    legal side of, 186–187
    resource referral, 189
    risks of, 183–184
    success story, 187–190

T

Teratospermia, defined, 27

Test tube baby, first, 19, 150–151, 283

Testes biopsy, 54, 156–157

Testicle problems, 28

Testicular cancer, 29, 55

Timed intercourse
    Clara and José's story, 82–83
    guidelines for, 79–80

Toxins, environmental, 85–88

Traditional surrogacy, 181

Treatment. *See* Complementary and
    alternative medicine; Medical
    treatment of females; Medical
    treatment of males

Triplets, 136, 257–258. *See also*
    Multiple births

Tubal disorders
    as cause of infertility, 21–22
    medical treatment for, 138, 153

Tubal ligation reversals, 138–139

Turner's syndrome, 32, 250

Twins, 136, 258. *See also* Multiple
    births

U

Ullmann, Liv, 279

Ultrasound exams
    for female, 60–61
    for male, 54

Underwear, men's, 30, 93

Urethra, defined, 6–7

Urethral opening, 29

Uterus
    abnormalities in, 137–138
    defined, 5
    examination of, 56

V

Vagina
    defined, 3
    illustrations of, 4, 5

Vaginal lubricants and douching,
    80–81

Varicoceles
    defined, 26–27
    exam for, 46
    treatment for, 142–143

Vas deferens, defined, 7, 27, 143

Vasectomy reversal, 143–144
Vasography, 54
Vegetarian women, 98–99
Venereal diseases, 14, 22, 27, 44,
    56, 138
Video display terminals (VDTs), 87
Vitex (chasteberry), 115
Vocabulary, helpful, 2–7, 27, 145
Vogel, Dr. Donna, 146

Wurn, Belinda, 122–124
Wurn, Larry, 122–124
Wurn technique, 122–124
Wynsome, Dr. Rebecca, 98–101,
    124–128

Y

Yoga, 235–239

W

Waiting-child adoption, 192–193, 195
Weight loss or gain, 91–92
Willadsen, Dr. Steen, 253
Wilson, Dr. Michael, 167

Z

ZIFT (zygote intrafallopian transfer)
    procedure, 71, 163, 165, 172
Zona pellucida, defined, 247
Zygote, defined, 145

About the Author

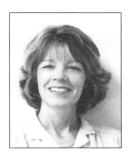

Theresa Foy DiGeronimo, M.Ed., is the author of numerous health books, including *New Hope for People with Lupus* and *New Hope for People with Fibromyalgia.* An adjunct professor teaching undergraduate and graduate writing courses at the William Paterson University of New Jersey, she lives in Hawthorne, New Jersey.

About the Medical Reviewer

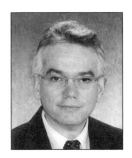

Paul R. Gindoff, M.D., is a professor of obstetrics and gynecology and the director of the Division of Reproductive Endocrinology, Fertility, and IVF at The George Washington University in Washington, D.C. He enjoys a prominent national and international reputation in reproductive endocrinology. Dr. Gindoff has conducted grant-sponsored clinical and basic research, as well as collaborative studies, at the National Institutes of Health where he served as an adjunct faculty member from 1988 to 1997.

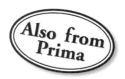
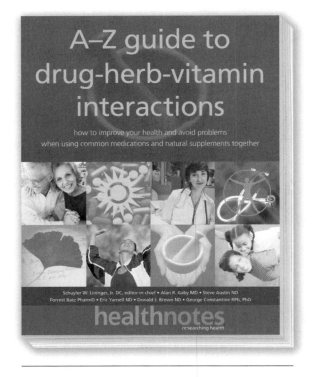